Leaving
Food
Behind

Price: Cdn $ 14.95
         U.S. $ 12.95

Leaving Food Behind

An Inspiring Personal Story of Recovery from
Bulimia, Starving, Overeating

Sheila Mather

Mather Publications
for Growth & Wellness Inc.

Published in 1997 by **Mather Publications for Growth and Wellness Inc.**
Nepean, ON, Canada

First Printing April 1997

Canadian Cataloguing in Publication Data:
Mather, Sheila Andrea, 1966—LEAVING FOOD BEHIND: an inspiring personal story of recovery from bulimia, starving and overeating

ISBN 0-9681812-1

    1. Mather, Sheila, 1966—Health. 2. Eating disorders—Patients—Biography. 3. Bulimia—Patients—Biography. I. Title.

I. Health, Personal I. Title

RC552.E18M378 1997 362.1'968526'0092 C97-900274-5

Copy Editor: Sherry Galey of Sherry Galey Editorial Services
Cover Design: DAX Communications Inc.
Typesetting: Lynn-Marie Nevin, Gorgias Communications

Printed in Canada

To my dear friend Howdy, to whom I am grateful beyond words, for his help throughout my entire recovery. To my sisters, Jen and Heidi, for their unwavering support. Thank you.

Table of Contents

Preface

ONE FALL AFTERNOON, I was in my apartment working away at my computer. I had just completed the outline of a book — this book. It was only an hour earlier that the thought of writing this book had let itself into my mind. Without hesitation I typed the words, they came so easily. There I was, looking at a book outline. I stared at it — in awe. I had no idea how I would ever write a book. I didn't know how to write, my English teachers could confirm that. Needless to say, I felt concerned but a moment later, and ever since, how I would write it didn't matter. From deep inside me, I knew that it would be written. I put my outline into an envelope and went to a friend's place to show him. With my mouth wide open, I looked at him excitedly and questioningly as he read it. Hanging on his every move, I gasped as he said, "this is marvelous. Of course you can write a book. If there is any way I can help, don't hesitate to ask." Filled with love and joy, I leapt into his arms — I was so very grateful for his support. I knew that I was about to write this book, somehow, someway.

Since that day, which was several months into my recovery, I've spent many hours alone at my computer, learning how to write, transforming my experience into words. Leaving Food Behind is my expression of how I saw the world, what I thought and how I felt — as a child, as a teenager, the years during my eating disorder, and ultimately, as an adult in recovery.

Although we all lived in the same house, my brothers and sisters didn't feel the same way about our experiences growing up as I did. I was (and still am) an extremely sensitive person who felt the slightest frown, smile, movement or word of everyone around me. I have come to appreciate that my perception of life is indeed different to that of many other people.

My journey of recovery was the most "feeling" experience of my life. Yes, it was painful as you will read, and yet, so beautiful. Through it, I became me, my soul, the person who is sharing these words with you. I know that a beautiful soul lies within each of us, just waiting to be released. Each human being has so much to offer the world. I offer these words to you with the fervent wish that my story will give you courage, hope and inspiration on your journey. God Bless you.

Sheila Mather

Since I am not a doctor, psychologist, or psychiatrist, etc., I made no recommendations on how to recover. I only knew what I needed to recover. I read many psychology books while I was in recovery, and some helped. (I read one book on bulimia when I was 23 years old, and because it described what I should eat, I did not gain from it.) Although I did not look for or receive assistance from an Eating Disorder Clinic, I know that helpful, exceptional clinics exist. For more information on Eating Disorders or to locate an Eating Disorder Clinic near you, you can contact:

In Canada: The National Eating Disorder Clinic — 1 (416) 340-4156 (Toronto, ON)

In the United States, consult your local telephone directory.

Introduction

Class was almost over and I felt a rush come over me. I was happy for the first time all day. I was going home to eat! I was absolutely invigorated. I could feel my heart pound and my mouth water. This time, I would have cake and butter tarts, yes, that would be perfect. All I cared about was eating, only eating. I was growing more excited by the moment. I left the classroom, in an almost full sprint. Now I felt desperate. I couldn't let anything stop me from eating. I felt as though I was running from a gruesome creature that would do me great harm if I didn't get home and fast. I had to eat — that would protect me. I climbed into my car and drove carelessly, speeding through traffic.

I stopped at the grocery store and bought the cake and butter tarts. When I got home, I ran into my apartment, locked the door, and left the world behind. I spread the food out onto the kitchen counter and chose my first serving. I plopped on the couch, turned on the television, and began to eat. It was as though someone had turned down the speed of a turntable — the speed of the world around me slowed from 78 r.p.m. to all but a stop. All sounds were muffled. My phone rang, and kept ringing. I was in a daze. Everything was okay, in fact more than okay. My fear of being hurt by that creature was gone — I was safe now. The food tasted so good. The pain dissolved. The anxiety vanished. The desperation disappeared. All those negatives floated away, like helium-filled balloons, into the sky. I felt absolutely wonderfully happy. Finally, I was at peace.

I went through that same process just about every day, sometimes as many as four times, for over 10 years. My eating disorder began when I was 15. My recovery began in 1992 when I was 25. I stopped binging, purging, starving and overeating in 1993. Although my eating disorder started when I was in grade 11, I felt the pain that drove me toward food for many years before that.

With food, I was able to control my pain and heartache. But, at 25, my pain seemed to boil over and I couldn't control it any longer. By then, I had lost my sense of humour, my desire to learn new things, my curiosity, and my desire to play. I felt as though I was drowning in pain. I was just existing, just trying to get through the day. I felt as though I was living beneath a black cloud that followed me everywhere.

When I embarked on my recovery, I began what was to be the most challenging, painful and rewarding time of my life. My recovery — which involved experiencing and understanding my past emotions — lasted more than four years. During the first three years I directed all my attention toward my personal well-being.

The first year, I cried often. I embraced my deepest, most painful emotions. It wasn't until the second year that I was able to make some sense of what was happening. It was then that I began to understand what caused me to reach for food. And though I cried less often, I still shed a great many tears. In the third year I began to make choices about my life. By the end of it, I had a clear picture of my past, present and my future. Beginning the fourth year and to the present, I felt invigorated, as though I were given a second chance in life. I was happy, truly happy, just to be here on earth.

Although I was actively binging, purging and starving until shortly before I began my recovery, I didn't think I had a problem with food. I knew that binging, purging and overeating was not right, but I thought that I could handle it. I had to handle it. I needed food. It helped me get through the rough times.

What happened to change all this? One day, I went for a walk down by the river. I stood close to the shore and watched the current flow. It was as though someone was shining a bright light on my life. Suddenly I saw my behaviour clearly. I had never before stopped to picture myself binging. I had no idea what I looked like, until now. I was shocked and disgusted. Before this, I couldn't, or rather wouldn't, let myself see what I was actually doing to myself, to my finances, to my integrity and to my life. But now, I could now see the reality in stark outline. I saw the way I had been stuffing food into my mouth rapidly and in great quantity.

I stood there, as if frozen. Although my feet were solidly planted on the earth, it seemed as if the ground was crumbling beneath me. I was scared. I didn't know what to do. I felt like I was in a deep black hole and couldn't find the opening. I looked up to the sky and pleaded: "Please help me!" Then I began to cry. I hadn't cried like that in a long, long time. Tears streamed down my face. I felt as though someone had pulled the plug on my feelings. Right then, right there, I knew that it was time to face my life. It was time to stop living in fear and pain. It was time to stop rushing home every night to binge. It was time to feel.

I went home that night and sat on my couch. I looked outside, but not at anything in particular. I was in a daze. I was totally exhausted. I was exhausted from the years of keeping my emotions inside, and from binging, purging, starving and overeating. Then, I heard a bird chirp. One had landed on my apartment balcony. It was singing — the pain and worries of the world had no place in its life. It was obviously happy. Then, somewhere deep inside me, I tapped into the knowledge that I would survive the months to come. I knew that one day, I too, would be happy. My recovery had begun.

The dictionary definition of "recovery" is *a regaining of something lost.*[1] I recovered myself. I regained my life. I rediscovered my feelings and emotions. I regained my joy and hope. I regained my zest for life. I recovered my heart and became a human being.

My process of recovery was an experience of learning how to get in touch with and allow myself to feel my emotions. I learned how to interpret, honour and express my feelings. By feeling, layers of protection, pain, and messages that had built up over the years and isolated me from real life, slowly disappeared. These were like protective layers of blankets enveloping me, layers that had come to suffocate me, instead of shield me from the cold.

Today, I don't eat when I'm not hungry. I would never have believed that I'd be able to eat only when hungry. I envied people who could respond to an offer of food with: "No thanks, I've already eaten." I'd wonder what having already eaten had to do with anything. Prior to my recovery, I could have eaten anytime.

During my recovery, I experienced the emotions of my past and my present and kindled my hopes for the future. In the movie *A Christmas Carol*, Ebenezer Scrooge was led into his past, present and future by three spirits. My recovery was a mental and emotional journey through my 25-year past. Unfortunately, my experience was much less clearly defined than that of Scrooge, but just as real. I had 25 years worth of painful and terrifying feelings inside me. At times, I felt overwhelmed with fear and insanity. The more emotions I felt, the more understanding, strength and compassion I gained.

During the time I was experiencing these emotions, I needed privacy. I stayed in my apartment most of the first year. I needed time and space from people, especially those who were apt to tell me how I should live. I didn't want to hear what was best for me. I stayed away from outside input. I had one friend with whom I shared my recovery. Alone, I was safe. I needed to be very safe to feel my emotions.

Although I was alone, I did have an outside source of strength. At times during my recovery, I could feel a presence near me (at least Scrooge could see his spirits, I thought I was going crazy). For the first while, I just brushed off this feeling because I wasn't the least religious. I didn't go

---

[1] Simon & Schuster, Inc, NEW WORLD DICTIONARY *of American English*, Third College Edition (New York, New York: Webster's New World Dictionaries, 1991), p 1122.

to church. I did believe that somewhere, far away, God existed. When I felt overwhelmed by my fears, I would read the poem *Footprints*.

> One night a man had a dream. He dreamed he was walking along the beach with the Lord. Across the sky flashed scenes from his life. For each scene, he noticed two sets of footprints in the sand: one belonging to him, and the other to the Lord. When the last scene of his life flashed before him, he looked back at the footprints in the sand. He noticed that many times along the path of his life there was only one set of footprints. He also noticed that it happened at the very lowest and saddest times in his life.
>
> This really bothered him and he questioned the Lord about it. "Lord, You said that once I decided to follow You, You'd walk with me all the way. But I have noticed that during the most troublesome times in my life, there is only one set of footprints. I don't understand why when I needed You most You would leave me."
>
> The Lord replied, "My son, My precious child, I love you and would never leave you. During your times of trial and suffering, when you see only one set of footprints, it was then that I carried you."
>
> —Author unknown

I loved that poem and by reading it often, I gained some much needed comfort, strength and faith to continue my recovery. At times, when I thought that I would die of sad feelings, I took great comfort in knowing that I wasn't alone. I knew that my times of trial and suffering had a purpose. I knew that they were necessary to take me to a better place. I knew that when I was strong enough, my two feet would be back on the ground in the sand.

There were many times I felt it was just too painful to continue and I often prayed that the pain would end. Yet, something inside me kept me feeling. I kept taking one step after another toward myself. I knew that if I didn't hang in there, I wouldn't recover. I knew that happiness awaited at the other end.

Throughout my recovery, people, books, songs and sights were available to me exactly when I needed them. I was very lucky to have had one very special friend who was there for me throughout my recovery. My friend offered his support, comfort, encouragement and very large ear. I am forever grateful to him.

I did not determine how, when or why I would recover. I did not enforce my recovery. I recovered because I stopped trying to control my eating. Prior to my recovery, I used to say: "I've got to stop eating like this," or "I'll quit binging and purging tomorrow." I thought that "I" was going to execute my recovery. Once I began my recovery, I allowed myself to binge and purge any time I felt the need. Very slowly, toward the end of the first year, my need to reach for food left me. One day, I realized that it had been two weeks since I had binged, purged, or overeaten.

I truly hope that by sharing my experience and recovery from bulimia, starving and overeating, that it can help others. Prior to my recovery, I felt so much pain that I didn't know what to do or where to turn. Food was my only relief, so I ate. By doing this, I shut out the rest of the world, and my pain increased. I felt even more lonely and isolated. Food couldn't take away my pain — eating was not the answer. I am so thrilled to have come to the place where, I know with all my heart, that *food can be left behind.*

By the end of the first year, I had begun to get to know and feel closer to myself. I began to see how beautifully the sun shone and the river flowed. I began to hear the birds chirping. I began to see a new, beautiful side to life, one that I had never known. It was even more glorious than I had imagined. At the end of that year, the storm cloud lifted. During the following year, without the need to binge and purge, I learned how I had been relating to the world (outside me) and how my heart felt (inside me).

When I began my recovery, I desperately wanted to know what caused my eating disorder. I wanted to understand how I got so out of control. What caused me to binge once I set my mind to it? What made me to eat when I wasn't hungry? Why did I never feel full or satisfied after eating a meal? Why did I obsess about what to eat, when to eat, and how much to eat? Why did I feel compelled to be slimmer and more attractive than other women? How would it ever end? I learned the answers to all those questions during my recovery. I feel grateful and blessed to be able to tell you about my experience.

One

MY
EATING
DISORDER

I t was early evening and I was getting ready to take a bath. The day had been exhausting, but these days, that's the way they all were. I had worked for nine hours and then exercised for two and a half. Before stepping into the bathtub, I stood before the mirror and stared at my legs in utter disgust. I felt betrayed by them. They were so big and ugly. I desperately wished I could change them. I was willing to try just about anything. I gripped the back of both legs and pulled at the skin and fat so I could see how they'd look if they were smaller. I liked what I saw. Earlier, I had exercised with a plastic bag over each leg to sweat away the fat. I had tried several slimming creams in the past — nothing worked. Feeling frustrated and powerless, I climbed into the bathtub and tried not to think about them. That didn't change anything, I still hated them. I turned my attention elsewhere. I looked down at my sore stomach and started yelling at it for being sore. Suddenly shaken by reality, I realized I was yelling at my own stomach!

That evening happened just months before I began my recovery. I hated my legs. I had never hated anything more. From my perspective at the time, they were the reason for all the pain in my life. They were the cause of all my feelings of my rejection and abandonment.

I couldn't acknowledge my legs as the part of my body that got me around or let me participate in sports. No way. They were fat and ugly and did nothing but make me miserable. I didn't perceive my stomach as part of me either. It was only after I heard myself yelling, that I realized, for the first time, how cruelly I had been treating my own living, breathing body. But then, I hadn't been treating any part of myself with love or kindness. My own body was foreign to me.

I felt so sad and so sorry. I rubbed my stomach. I looked at my legs and said I was sorry. How could I have been so cruel? I felt like a stranger in my own skin. How had I become so mentally and emotionally split, so estranged from my own body?

I was now 25 years old. I had been split like this for many years. Thinking back, I can't recall a time since I was seven that I really acknowledged my body as mine. By the time my eating disorder began at age 15, I had lost any awareness that I lived in my body. Over the next 10 years, I treated my body, as well as my mind and my emotions, as though they belonged to someone else.

The dictionary definition of "addiction" is *to give (oneself) up (to some strong habit), usually in the passive.*[1] I had *given up* myself. Until then, I had not been aware of what I had been doing. I was shocked to hear myself yell at my own body. I actually hated a part of myself. I had completely rejected myself. I had given up on myself mentally, physically and emotionally. I was convinced I was stupid, that I was ugly and overweight, and that my emotions were shameful and disgusting. Having slim legs meant more to me than treating myself with love, respect and care. I had *given up* myself in every way.

I had given up nourishing my body with food. I starved and then purged most of what I did eat. Then, taking it to the other extreme, I placed an unbelievable amount of stress on my digestive system by overeating. On many a weekend I would eat six meals within the span of a couple of hours. I put my health in grave jeopardy.

I had given up my desire to eat what I wanted. I placed tight restrictions on what I ate. I put my fear of gaining weight before my own desires. The evening I yelled at my sore stomach, I had starved for the previous three days and then binged that day. No wonder my stomach was sore!

I had given up caring for my body. I didn't touch it, rub it or apply cream to it. I didn't get enough sleep or drink enough water. All I cared about was making it slim. My body was an object that was either too fat or not right in some other way. Every time I looked at it, I looked at it objectively, rating it, as I thought someone else would. I didn't think about the fact that I was breathing with it, or doing anything with it. I did things to it.

I showed my body no mercy. I exercised so that it would look better, not so that I would feel good. Some of the exercises I put my body through were downright cruel. I would push my body well beyond its capacity. Near exhaustion, after a ten-mile run, I would force myself to run a few more miles. I would run too fast and bike too hard. I didn't care how I felt. Out in public, I exercised in order to be seen as athletic, attractive and desirable.

I had given up my emotions. I would simply not allow myself to feel things, especially pain. The only time I allowed myself to feel joy or pain was when I ate, the only time I felt safe enough. I had abandoned (given up) my heart. No wonder I felt as though I didn't belong to anything! I didn't allow my heart to belong to me. I felt as though I had no foundation.

---

[1]Simon & Schuster, Inc., *NEW WORLD DICTIONARY of American English*, Third College Edition (New York, New York: Webster's New World Dictionaries, 1991), p 15.

I was completely disconnected and I felt a desperate need to connect. I badly needed a foundation and didn't understand why I didn't have one. It was only when I ate that I felt grounded, but food could never be the foundation I truly needed. What I sorely needed to do, was to reconnect with my body, mind and emotions.

My life was incomplete and utter "disorder" (*lack of order, confusion*[2]). My list of priorities were completely mixed up. Food was at the top, other people were next and I was at the bottom. Food had replaced me as the central theme and foundation of my life. Other people's thoughts, feelings, preferences and judgments were much more important than my own.

I tried to instill order by controlling my body and my eating. No one could tell me how much to eat. I could fight back. I could show everyone else and myself who was in charge. By starving myself and losing weight, I could convince myself I was in control. I had accomplished something. I stood tall and felt powerful.

Unfortunately, the more control I tried to exert, the more disordered my life became. The more I focused on my body size and food intake, the less I focused on my friends, family, parties, playing guitar and other parts of my life. After a while, those things fell away and I eventually lost them. I became obsessed with control, "obsessed" (*to haunt or trouble in mind, esp. to an abnormal degree, to preoccupy greatly*[3]) with my body size and my food intake. By my early twenties, nothing mattered to me more than my weight. I must have weighed myself five to ten times a day. I probably looked at myself in the mirror at least 20 times. I would spend hours in front of the mirror, examining every ugly inch, and wanting to change it all.

I was obsessed with how much I ate, what kind of food I ate, and how to lose more weight. I read every diet book on the market. I knew a lot about food, especially which foods were highest in calories and fat. I knew that my body began to digest sugar 30 seconds after I put it into my mouth. I knew that it takes longer to digest proteins and complex carbohydrates than simple sugars. When I binged, and intended to purge, I would eat sugars last. I didn't want to digest any food. I was certain that all my pain and worries would be gone if I were slim. I felt safe when my stomach was empty, safe that I wasn't gaining weight.

Many of you are probably familiar with the terms *anorexia nervosa* and *bulimia*. For those who aren't, I include here the definitions of these eating disorders taken from the American Psychiatric Association's Diagnostic and Statistical Manual of Mental Disorders, Fourth Edition (DSM IV).

---

[2]Simon & Schuster Inc., p 395.
[3]Simon & Schuster, Inc., p 936.

Anorexia Nervosa[4] is characterized by a refusal to maintain a minimally normal body weight. *Bulimia Nervosa*[5] is characterized by repeated episodes of binge eating followed by inappropriate compensatory behaviours such as self-induced vomiting; misuse of laxatives, diuretics, or other medications; fasting; or excessive exercise.

Although *Compulsive Overeating* is not listed in the DSM IV, I believe that it is also an eating disorder. I define *Compulsive Overeating* as characterized by the compulsion to eat whether or not a person is experiencing physical hunger. Eating may be continued to the point of severe abdominal discomfort. I believe that food allergies (fixed, cyclic or addictive) may contribute to the obsessive nature of a food addiction as well.

I always cringe when I hear a doctor or someone else describe a human being as a *bulimic*. To me, that label is so shaming. One of the reasons I didn't seek help from the medical profession was precisely because I was carrying enough shame for 10 people. I couldn't stand to listen to someone define me by a clause or paragraph in a textbook. I had an eating disorder. I knew that. I didn't want or need anyone to read aloud the gruesome details of how I was living my life.[6]

There is no question that my eating was extremely disordered. I had long before lost the natural feeling of being hungry or full. I overate or I starved. My head dictated what went into my stomach. I ate while driving, in between classes at school, on a coffee break at work, while watching television, and when I went out with friends. Most often, I ate when I was anxious, tense, sad, and alone. I felt comforted by food. I ate even when I was physically satisfied or nourished. I ate until I could eat no more. My stomach would be so stuffed with food that I couldn't move, yet I longed for just one more bite. I also used to starve myself, sometimes for as long as three days, eating only a few pieces of bread and a little fruit.

When I got so hungry that I couldn't stand it, I would eat enough for five days. I would stuff food into my mouth like a wild animal. After about two months, I learned to purge after the binges. But I still starved

---

[4]American Psychiatric Association. *Diagnostic and Statistical Manual of Mental Disorders,* Fourth Edition. Washington, D.C., American Psychiatric Association, 1994, p. 539.
[5]American Psychiatric Association, p 539.
[6]A year after I had recovered, I had occasion to speak with a professional who was treating four patients who had bulimia. He had been quite graciously describing the enigma he felt surrounded the cause of eating disorders. After some time, he began to describe, with great disgust, how one of his patients had resumed binging after one year of abstinence. "I don't understand bulimics!" he exclaimed. I was mortified. I was also grateful that I hadn't chosen to get help from the professional community. I now know that helpful professionals do exist.

as long as I could, until I couldn't take it one more moment and then I'd binge. I was totally unaware of the game I was playing with myself. I would starve myself to punish myself for being weak and giving in to food again. The more food I binged on, the harsher the penalty I would impose — the longer the period I'd make myself starve.

When I could endure the pain of purging, I was bulimic. I ate until I could take in no more, and then purge by putting my finger down my throat. I became quite adept at it. I rarely purged outside my own home. When I could sustain the agony of it, I would starve myself all day and then binge at night. I purged after most binges. However, there was a period when I didn't purge because I couldn't stand the physical pain and I stopped. When I gained the inevitable weight, I'd force myself to start purging again.

I didn't binge after eating any particular food. I have heard that a "trigger food" can bring on a binge. Not for me. I didn't binge because of a physical need. However, I usually purged when I ate a sweet or high fat "fattening food" because I believed I would gain weight if I didn't.

Food had long since lost its significance as a substance that nourished me and gave me energy. It was a substance that I could control, if taken in limited enough quantitites it could make me look beautiful, and if overeaten, it could make me ugly.

I knew that I had to be inflicting harm on my body, but I didn't care. I binged, purged, overate and starved anyway. However, so you can be aware of what can happen , these are some potential side-effects. Many of the physical signs and symptoms of *Anorexia Nervosa* are attributable to starvation. In addition to amenorrhea, there may be complaints of constipation, abdominal pain, cold intolerance, lethargy and excess energy. The most obvious finding on physical examination is emaciation. There may also be significant hypotension, hypothermia and skin dryness. Recurring vomiting can eventually lead to a significant and permanent loss of dental enamel.[7]

Menstrual irregularity or amenorrhea sometimes occurs among females with *Bulimia Nervosa*; whether such disturbances are related to weight fluctuations, to nutritional deficiencies, or to emotional stress is uncertain. Rare, but potentially fatal, complications include esophageal tears, gastric rupture and cardiac arrhythmias.[8]

I had my share of side-effects.When I first lost weight, at age 15, I weighed 113 pounds. For the next two years, I weighed between 113 and

---

[7]American Psychiatric Association. *Diagnostic and Statistical Manual of Mental Disorders,* Fourth Edition. Washington, D.C., American Psychiatric Association, 1994, p. 542.
[8]American Psychiatric Association. *Diagnostic and Statistical Manual of Mental Disorders,* Fourth Edition. Washington, D.C., American Psychiatric Association, 1994, p. 548.

115 pounds. I felt great. I had attained my ulimate goal — losing weight. I stood 5' 8 3/4 inches tall, weighed 113 pounds and wore a size five — loosely. I was skinny! Yet every time I looked in the mirror, I saw a place on my body that I thought should be smaller. I always wanted to lose five more pounds. I remember stepping on the scale when it read 113 pounds and thinking: "Okay, now if I can just lose five more!" I had no idea of what I was doing to myself. I only knew that I had to be slim, and had to continue to lose weight.

My gums were receding. At 18, the dentist told me that I had the gums of a 30- year-old, and they were only going to get worse if I didn't start to floss. Fortunately for me, he had no idea that the condition of my gums had nothing to do with a failure to floss. However, at that point, nothing could have stopped me from binging and purging. My bulimia lasted for another seven years.

I developed a digestive tract disorder which prevented me from digesting many foods. My hair became very dry and the ends split; I had dark circles under my eyes; and my face would swell up for a good six hours after purging. My weekly weight fluctuations slowed my metabolism and made me feel constantly fatigued. My period was irregular and almost nonexistent. Most obviously, purging had left bruises that ran across my stomach at my abdominal sphincter. I was in bad shape, and getting worse, but I continued binging, purging, starving and overeating.

I was playing an all-or-nothing game with myself. I would taunt myself with thoughts of butter tarts and cake and then tell myself: "Forget it, you're not touching any of it." I would deny myself until I couldn't stand it one more moment, then I would snap back like an overextended elastic, and binge. Binging was failing. Starving was winning the game of control. My life was about controlling every thing and everyone in it. I had given up all that was enjoyable in my life. I controlled and restricted my mind, body and emotions.

All I cared about now was getting away from the cruel tyrant inside of me who was driving me to such extremes. I didn't know what was possessing me to do such terrible things to myself. I felt terrified about what was happening to me. I felt as though I was going insane. I was totally out of control. And I hated it. I hated food. I hated my body. And I especially hated me.

Two

GUILT

I was walking by the display window of an accessory store when I saw the most gorgeous beige Italian leather purse. I decided to go inside. Upon taking a closer look, I loved it even more. It was expensive, but worth the price. Although I desperately wanted that beautiful purse, I walked out of the store, without it. I felt sad, as though I had just been told by parent that we couldn't afford it. I had enough money, but I couldn't bring myself to spend it on a purse. There were more important necessities to buy.

I walked home feeling frustrated and confused because I would not buy myself that purse. No, part of me knew I had to be more practical. I wasn't worthy of having such an exquisite purse. I had to make sure everyone else was taken care of first. I felt a little better. I was almost home when I realized that I could buy the purse for my sister. She'd love it, and she needed a new purse anyway. I went right back to the store and bought the purse for her. After all, she deserved it more than I did.

I was 19. By this time, I had been binging and purging for four years. I knew how to restrict my food intake, as well as all my other desires. I would never have bought that purse for myself — it would have made me feel too "guilty." (*Guilt is a painful feeling of self-reproach resulting from a belief that one has done something wrong or immoral.*[1]) I could not justify spending money on such an unnecessary, luxurious purchase. Had I bought it for myself, I would have driven myself crazy thinking about all the ways I could have spent the money more wisely and responsibly. I needed nylons, face cream, bed sheets and dish cloths. I had no trouble buying gifts, however. I never felt guilty spending money on other people. I just couldn't spend money on myself — I wasn't worth it. I felt selfish for even wanting that purse.

For years, growing up in my home, I felt responsible for what happened to my family. (No one ever told me that I was, I just felt that way.)

---

[1] Simon & Schuster, Inc., p 600.

I felt responsible when anyone in my family experienced pain. Even though I was just a kid, I felt as though it was up to me to make sure that my brothers, sisters and parents were happy. I couldn't stand the thought that they might be feeling the same horrible sadness that I felt. No way, it was my role to prevent that from ever happening.

One evening, my family went to McDonald's for dinner. I told my brothers and sisters exactly what to eat. I felt it was my job to make sure that they didn't order anything too expensive. I had to conserve our family's money. I tried to do that every time we went out. When I succeeded, I felt relieved. When I failed, I would feel guilty.

I felt very guilty for wanting or needing anything for myself. It seemed to me that satisfying a want or need would always be at the expense of others. Like the expensive purse I couldn't buy, I couldn't order an expensive restaurant meal. I would never ask for anything unless I was positive that no one would suffer if I received it. I hated receiving gifts and told people not to buy me things.

I always put the needs and wants of others before my own. I longed to take care of myself but I couldn't bare the guilt. In my mind, someone else had to lose if I gained, so I took care of others instead. I did many things for others, especially things I wanted to do for myself. I would buy something for someone else — something I wanted — like the purse for my sister. I wanted others to feel like they were being taken care of, the same way that I wanted to be.

By putting other people's needs first, I abandoned my own. I felt as though no one was looking out for me. I would feel hurt and upset, and not know why. While I was doing things for others, I could not hear my own voice scream: "Hey! What about me?" I needed me. I needed my own help, and I wasn't there for myself.

I tried to be super-responsible at home. While I was in high school, I played sports every day after school so I wasn't at home very often, but when I was, I cleaned the house, baked desserts and did as much as I could for my family. I felt that I was simply fulfilling my responsibilities. I was told that I was "a thoughtful young lady who put other people first." I loved getting that recognition.

I couldn't stand to sit by and allow someone to struggle with a problem. I would immediately jump in and take over. I felt completely responsible for solving it. It never even occurred to me that maybe, just maybe, I had nothing to do with it! I never imagined that a person might be experiencing a problem so they could learn to solve it, and grow stronger, wiser and happier. I've never really felt good when anyone took over and solved my problem. I felt no sense of accomplishment nor did I learn anything. I only learned that I wasn't capable of solving my problems myself.

I hated confrontations! To me, an argument was a clear example of my failure. I wanted everyone to be happy. Growing up, I frequently took the blame for things that happened between my brothers and sisters, just to keep peace in the family. One evening, my father gathered my two brothers and two sisters together for a meeting. The topic was stolen money. Someone was missing a couple of dollars from their piggy bank. I couldn't stand the tension, so I confessed to taking it. I hadn't stolen it, but by confessing, I brought an end to that unhappy situation. On the other hand, when I really did do something wrong, I wouldn't admit it because I was too afraid of being rejected.

I tried to read minds, and I went to great lengths to anticipate what people were thinking and feeling, and try to predict their needs and wants. When I did that, I was better able to satisfy their needs, and I received even more praise for being so perceptive and sensitive. I always said things I thought others wanted to hear. I rarely disagreed with people because I didn't want anyone to feel insulted or stupid.

To avoid hurting peoples' feelings, I made commitments I didn't want to make; I didn't have the guts to say no. However, once I made an un-wanted commitment, I'd feel resentful for giving up my time yet again. Then I'd feel guilty for feeling resentful. I'd also go out with people I didn't enjoy being with. I did many things I didn't want to do. Yet, I never felt guilty for hurting myself instead. I thought I could handle it.

I felt guilty for having things, for doing things, for trying things, for showing confidence. I would hear remarks like: "Who do you think you are?"; "What makes you think that you can do that?"; "How in the world did you afford that?"; "You'll end up paying for it in the end"; and "How could you be so selfish?" There were so many more.

I never wanted anyone to be envious of me. I felt guilty for being pretty, having nice hair and clothes, being able to sing, working at an enjoyable job, making money or getting a promotion. I felt guilty when I was given an opportunity and someone else wasn't. I would often ruin or downgrade my opportunities so that this wouldn't happen.

I worked at many jobs I didn't enjoy. I believed that a job was supposed to be boring, gruelling, and full of drudgery. At one point I left one job to work at another, which offered less security, but much more personal satisfaction. At the time, people said things like: "Must be nice"; "Are you ever lucky"; and "I can't believe you left a stable, secure income to do this." I felt as though they were telling me: "I'm miserable, so you should be too." I felt guilty when I enjoyed my work while others hated theirs.

I felt so guilty about needing or wanting something that I justified my every move beforehand to prove that my needs and wants were valid. I felt compelled to justify everything I did, said and felt. I began most of my sentences with: "I just…" — as in "I just want…"; "I just thought…" or "I just needed…" and complete each sentence with a lengthy explanation. If I justified all my feelings, thoughts and actions I could reduce the chance for shame, judgment, rejection or guilt.

Although I tried as hard as I could, but I couldn't possibly ensure that everyone was happy all of the time. Unfortunately, I didn't know that at the time. I thought that, if they weren't, it was my fault — that I had failed to live up to my responsibilities. When people were feeling sad or experiencing hardships, I felt like I was the real failure. I felt incredible shame.

****

Three

****

SHAME

I couldn't take another bite. I stood up, dizzy with nausea and pain. My stomach was distended like a balloon. I had eaten so much I could barely move. I stumbled past the empty boxes and wrappers that covered the kitchen counter. When I reached the bathroom, I looked at myself in the mirror with utter disgust. I had done it again — binged. I couldn't believe it. I felt so weak, so pathetic, and so shameful. This meant that I'd have to go through the pain of purging again. I felt too sick to wait another moment. I got down on my knees and purged and purged. The more food I got rid of, the more relieved I felt. I wouldn't stop until I had gotten rid of every last bit. It was all so disgusting. When I had finished, I looked at myself in the mirror again. I was completely exhausted and so very ashamed.

I knew there was something wrong with me, there had to be. A good person wouldn't binge on enormous amounts of food, and then purge. I was absolutely disgusted by this behaviour — and I was doing it! I felt "shame" right down to my core. (*Shame is an emotion caused by a strong sense of guilt, embarrassment, unworthiness, or disgrace*[1]).

I didn't just feel shame as an emotion, I experienced myself as shameful. Back then, I didn't recognize that my thoughts and feelings are not me — that who I am is distinct from what I think and how I feel. All I could see was a guilty, embarrassing, unworthy and disgraceful person. I didn't just *feel* stupid and unworthy of being loved, I genuinely believed I *was* stupid and unworthy of being loved.

I felt shame for so many things — for burdening my parents, requiring them forego satisfying their needs in favour of mine. I got the grossest "yuck" feeling in the pit of my stomach any time I even considered my needs or wants. I felt unworthy of care, time, effort and attention. I truly believed I didn't deserve to be fed, given nice gifts, have good, trustworthy

---

[1]Simon & Schuster, Inc., p 600.

friends or be offered career opportunities. I didn't deserve to be happy, to succeed, to do what I wanted, or feel good about myself.

Most of all, I had no doubt that I didn't deserve to be loved as I was. I believed that if I was ever to be loved by someone, it would be up to me to make it happen. I would have to change the way I was and that meant losing weight.

There were so many things I didn't deserve. I didn't deserve to eat food I enjoyed — things like cookies, cakes (especially cheesecake), sloppy hamburgers, french fries, chicken wings (with skin!), fried zucchini sticks and creamy sauces. I rarely kept these foods down because I didn't want to gain weight. I was convinced that I was the only person in the world who couldn't eat these foods without putting on the pounds. So, I purged. To me, weight gain was the punishment for enjoying these foods.

I felt stupid, unable to follow through on tasks, too weak to excel at anything. I felt downright useless, incapable of learning or applying skills successfully. I tried many things but mastered none. I was convinced that although I was a good athlete, I could never attain the level of excellence required to be a professional. Even though I was a good basketball and tennis player, I always fell short of being great.

I felt unappreciated. I did so much for people and received so little gratitude in return. Although I was hurt by this, deep down I wasn't surprised because I didn't really deserve it anyway. I remember once asking a friend to watch a video of a fashion show I was in. When he didn't, I was wounded, but this only confirmed my sense that I wasn't worthy of his time. Time was precious, and it was presumptuous of me to ask others for some of theirs. I just wasn't worth it.

I was sure that other people could see my shamefulness. If they didn't see it immediately, they would eventually. I constantly worried about what others thought of me. I tried to conceal my shame from the eyes of the world. Every time I felt stupid, dumb, incapable, worthless or uncoordinated, I felt ashamed. Every time I made a mistake, I felt ashamed.

To lessen my shamefulness, I did everything I could to become the embodiment of what others wanted — a pretty, slim, happy, kindhearted young woman. I said all the things I was supposed to say. I did everything I was supposed to do. I was like an actress. I learned how to act by observing how movie actresses played their roles. I used to think: "I could do that." I was right. I was doing it.

I was always performing. Acting was fun. It protected me like a suit of armour and allowed me to reveal very little of my true self. If a person rejected my words or actions, I knew it wasn't a rejection of me. I figured out which roles people liked best by their reactions. When I received positive feedback and recognition for something, I felt wonderful and would repeat it. My roles were all in an attempt to gain a response from my audience.

This life of role-playing was hard work! (Later, after my recovery, people were shocked to hear what had actually been going on in my life during this period. Nobody could believe that there had been anything wrong. My acting had fooled them completely!)

I rarely expressed my own ideas, opinions or desires, especially when I perceived that someone might disagree. I wouldn't acknowledge many wonderful ideas because they got a negative reaction when I shared them. I stopped singing when people laughed. I stopped playing guitar because it was too noisy. As I grew up, I became less and less me, and more and more of what others wanted me to be. I saw my creative expressions as poisonous. Expressing myself got me yelled at or rejected. I believed that if I ever let myself show my true self, I'd never be loved.

I strived to be perfect — always. I figured if I was perfect, I couldn't be rejected. I longed for the perfect body and the most beautiful face. I wanted to be the best at everything I tried. I wanted to have the perfect house, the perfect car, the perfect job, the perfect clothes, etc. I couldn't stand it if my house was a mess when someone came to visit. I wanted to say the "right" thing, stand the "right" way, be associated with the "right" people, and wear the "right" clothes. I struggled to appear perfect on the outside so that no one would ever see how shameful I was on the inside.

I tried to do everything perfectly to avoid criticism. I'd carefully observe what other kids were punished for and resolve never to make the same mistakes. I tried not to do anything that would cause others to think badly of me. I never repeated actions that provoked criticism or punishment. In later years, when I did something that brought criticism, I felt a twinge of the familiar pain of shame.

I had a hard time learning something for the first time because I was convinced I wouldn't be able to do it perfectly. I would become so anxious, even angry, before I was about to do something if I wasn't sure I could do it perfectly. I had to win at everything. When I didn't, I felt like more of a loser, even more shameful. Losing just confirmed that I didn't have enough talent or brains to accomplish something. Each time I failed or lost, I heard the voice in my head that said: "See, I knew you couldn't do it." When I won, the shame would disappear.

The problem was that I could never find out what the "perfect" or "right" thing was. I continually failed in my quest to achieve perfection.

I craved attention and desperately wanted to be the light of everyone's eyes. I wanted to "wow" people, especially men. One day, when I was ten, I was practising gymnastics in the basement of our house. I fantasized that I was on a stage and the boy across the street was watching me. I could do no wrong. He loved me. He thought that I was the most beautiful, talented, wonderful girl he had ever seen. I had "wowed" him. I didn't feel as shameful then.

I preferred to be around people who weren't sure of themselves. I felt very uncomfortable, inferior and worthless around confident people. I was afraid they would see through me and my shame. To raise my own self-worth, I gossiped, criticized and ridiculed other people. I mentally stepped on people to rise above my shame. Throughout my school years, my girlfriends and I would gossip for hours. Of course, we directed our sternest judgment toward the girls who were pretty, smart and popular. Although I felt better about myself when I put someone else down, after awhile, I'd feel guilty about it. And I sure hated it when people gossiped about me.

The truth is, I judged myself the harshest of all. I would condemn myself many times a day. If I fumbled with the dishes, I'd scold: "Are you ever clumsy!"; or, "Pay attention!"; or "Don't be so stupid!" I'd call myself a "fat slob" and a "failure," especially after binging or eating fattening food. I've even gone so far to hit myself in the face to show utter contempt toward myself for being stupid and unattractive. I judged myself with cruel, hurtful thoughts — thoughts that could crush even the toughest of egos.

I took everything personally. When someone didn't listen to me, I assumed it was because I wasn't worth listening to. When someone told me that I wasn't suited for a job, I knew it was because I wasn't worthy of the position. When I wasn't chosen to be in a fashion show, it was because I wasn't slim enough. When a driver passed me, it was because I was driving too slowly. When I was in a car accident, it was because I was a bad driver. I believed that I was always at fault. This led me to respond defensively to everyone and everything. If someone commented that my lunch was large, I would take their observation as a reproach for eating too much. I would justify the size of my lunch and prove that it was low in calories and fat. I didn't receive any remarks about food as complimentary.

I lived a shame-ridden, fearful and painful life. I longed to live but I felt like I was slowly dying. I lived to hide my shamefulness from others, to be worthy of being loved even when I knew that I was shameful. I was living a life on the run, one step ahead of my shame. I was terrified of my shame. I was terrified, period.

My body weight had become the symbol of my shame. I measured my shame by the number on my scale. I stepped on my shame scale and felt less shame when my weight was low; more shame when it was high. However, shame was always present. By this time, I had learned that the one sure way to be acceptable and not rejected was to be slim. I was complimented when I was slim, rejected when I wasn't. (Chapter 12 describes how I perceive the importance of appearance in our culture.)

My solution: lose the weight, lose the shame. The problem was that losing weight didn't make the shame go away. I still felt unworthy of love. I still felt as incapable as ever. I was confused. The only solution I had wasn't working. My shame was still there. So I tried even harder to lose weight. I was more determined than ever.

At 113 pounds, I still felt terrible. I wanted to weigh 110. I was on a downhill spiral and way out of control. Thankfully, I couldn't continue to starve myself. I was headed toward a dangerously unhealthy weight — and fast.

****
Four
****

FEAR

I t was the middle of the night and I must have been in the middle of a dream. I was very disoriented. Arising from my daze, I realized that I was alone in bed. A dart of pain shot through my body. In the darkness, alone with my teddy bear, I felt so sad, so empty, so alone and so afraid. I curled up in a little ball and pulled my comforter over my head. I desperately wanted to retreat into myself somehow. I wanted to find safety inside my shell. I lived in fear that one day, this pain would catch me and swallow me up. I couldn't imagine surviving it. I knew that I had to stay one step ahead of this pain — always.

I was scared of life and everything in it, although I didn't realize it at the time. I knew only that I was extremely anxious, but I didn't know why. Fear was so much a part of my life that its absence would have created even more fear. "Fear" is *a feeling of anxiety and agitation caused by the presence or nearness of danger, evil, pain, etc.; dread; terror; fright; apprehension*[1]. I had never known life without it.

It was only after I began my recovery that I realized how completely fear had driven my life. There had been no real threats, just the usual stresses of life, nothing extraordinary. Despite that, I was overwhelmed by fear. Everything, and I mean everything, scared me. I felt as though a big black cloud hung over me, ready to strike lightning at any time. I feared that the rug would be pulled out from under me at any time. Everything, the spoken word, a telephone call or even a letter, could frighten me. I was petrified, certain that disaster was inevitable, especially when I least expected it. So, I was always alert and ready; I never let my guard down. I thought I was being very wise to be so well prepared.

I responded to many situations by feeling at least a slight twinge of fear, but more often it was full-blown panic. Panic felt like a sudden overwhelming chill pulsing throughout my body from the middle of my chest. When I was in its grip, I couldn't see clearly or do anything rational. I felt

---

[1]Simon & Schuster, Inc., p 495.

stunned. I panicked when my boss called me up to his office, when I got a letter from the bank, when I saw a police car. I was sure the worst was about to happen — the boss would fire me, the bank would cancel my credit, and the police would remove my driver's licence. I could panic anywhere, any place and anytime, I wasn't picky. When my fears didn't materialize, I felt as though I'd barely escaped certain catastrophe.

One day, I was reading a book called *You'll See It When You Believe It*[2] by Wayne Dyer. In it, the author describes how important it is to "embrace your fears." At the time, my reaction was: "Ha, forget it!" The last thing I wanted to do was "hug" those terribly horrifying things, fears.

That was before my recovery. Soon after it began, when I felt courageous enough, I wrote about and talked about some of my fears. At first, it was very difficult because some of the people I chose to share my fears with were not very understanding. One of them laughed and another told me I was "being ridiculous", "don't worry about that" and "you have nothing to be afraid of." This didn't help at all. I didn't need to hear that my fears were invalid, wrong, stupid or ridiculous, however imaginary they may have been. They were very real to me. I didn't need to be shamed. I never talked to those people again about my fears.

I found it challenging to continue to face my fears, with or without the help of other people. Fear was ingrained in my thoughts. Back then, I didn't recognize a fear as just a "thought," and I didn't know that my thoughts might not be real. They were terrifyingly real to me. I was sure they could take form at any moment. I had a very active imagination — I could picture the most gruesome and horrific scenarios. Given that, embracing my fear seemed completely out of the question.

I was fortunate to have one friend who supported and validated my feelings. I felt safe enough to talk to him about my fears and always felt better afterward. Alone, without the comfort of someone who cared, I would never have faced my fears. I would confide to him the horrendous things I was sure would befall me.

One day, my boss asked to see me the next day. I responded with utter panic. That evening, I called my friend and confessed that I was terrified I was going to be fired. Then I wouldn't have a job, I wouldn't be able to support myself and I'd be on the street, helpless and alone! Wow! After I divulged this, I couldn't believe what I just said. I had no idea that I was so terrified.

---

[2]Dr. Wayne W. Dyre, *You'll See It When You Believe It*, (New York, New York: Avon Books, 1989). (Although embracing my fears terrified me at the time, when I was ready, I did hug my fears. I loved the book by Wayne Dyre.)

My friend helped me take a closer look at the reality of the situation. I was able to acknowledge that losing my job would create pressure, but it was nothing I couldn't handle. I would look for another job and I was quite capable of finding one. I wouldn't have to live on the street, alone and helpless. I had never before walked through my fear like that. I was happy and very relieved. (It turned out that my boss wanted to see me in order to tell me what a wonderful job I had been doing!)

Writing and talking about my fears and their consequences made me come face-to-face with the one great fear that was at the heart of all the rest. *I was afraid of being abandoned.* I believed that if I were abandoned I would be alone and unable to survive. I went crazy when someone abandoned me physically by ending a relationship, or emotionally, by not listening to me or validating my feelings. My jealousy was also linked to my fear of abandonment.

My fear of abandonment spawned all my other fears.

- *Fear of rejection* — I wanted approval and acceptance from everyone, even strangers or mere acquaintances. I needed everyone to like and accept me.
- *Fear of being alone* — I was so scared of being alone because I thought isolation meant death. I thought I needed to be taken care of by someone else.
- *Fear of being left out* — I got really upset at people when they didn't include me in an activity. If I were left out, I thought I'd be forgotten and be left alone.
- *Fear of being left behind* — I thought I would die if I were left behind.
- *Fear of dying* — I was afraid of dying, particularly in a plane crash, by drowning or in a fire. I couldn't stand the thought of a tragic death. Then I'd been completely alone. I hated to hear about people who were beaten and left for dead — my worst nightmare.
- *Fear of trusting* — I was sure that if I trusted, I would experience pain. I would not allow myself to be vulnerable or trust.
- *Fear of God* — I figured God probably existed, but He was far, far away. I was certain that I had sinned enough in my life to warrant a major punishment from God. I didn't know who God was or what He was about. I was afraid of what His will might be. No way was I about to surrender my will or control of my life to Him.
- *Fear of not being safe/protected* — I wanted my mother to be with me. I wanted my mother and only my mother to protect me, no one else would do. Although I had lived without my mother for many years since she left the family, I yearned for the safety I felt with her.
- *Fear of the unknown* — Before I became involved in anything, I needed to know what was going to happen and what the outcome would be.

I felt very apprehensive when I couldn't predict the future. I had to know whether I would survive.

- *Fear of feeling my shame* — When I felt shame, I felt overwhelming fear, anxiety and absolute utter craziness. I would panic. It was as though I was reliving my abandonment. I believed that I had been abandoned and left alone because I was so shameful.

- *Fear of not being perfect/of being exposed* — I was terrified that people would find out I wasn't perfect, wasn't smart, wasn't a great tennis player, wasn't a great person. I was afraid that people would see right through me and my shame would be exposed.

- *Fear of criticism* — When someone was critical of me, I felt shameful. I was positive they were right, regardless of whether or not their criticism was valid.

- *Fear of losing* — I had to win. I was extremely competitive. Losing could mean being rejected. Losing meant being less interesting, pretty, intelligent, strong or lovable. I had to be the best. I had to outdo others. I couldn't stand it when a man I cared about was attracted to other women.

- *Fear of being judged* — I hated to be judged because I knew that I would be seen as unworthy of love, admiration or acceptance. I was afraid of being punished for being so terrible.

- *Fear of failing* — I was so afraid that I wouldn't be loved if I were a failure. Since I believed I was a failure, I did fail many of the things I tried. I failed before I even began. Failing confirmed my shame and fuelled my fear.

- *Fear of expressing how I really felt* — I was certain that I would be rejected, ridiculed and hurt if I vocalized how I really felt. As well, I was afraid if I hurt someone else's feelings, they would reject me.

- *Fear of being overweight* — I dreaded the possibility of being overweight. I was afraid people would reject me if I were fat.

- *Fear of not being fed* — I would eat even when I wasn't hungry because I didn't know when I'd have my next meal. I feared not being able to eat when I was hungry.

- *Fear of being trapped* — I had an enormous need to be free. Free of what, I don't know. I often felt trapped in a situation that I had committed to. I feared that I'd hate to be where I was, what I was doing or who I was with. I needed to feel safe and if I couldn't be, then I needed to be able to get out of the situation.

- *Fear of being taken advantage of* — When someone did something thoughtful for me, I always wondered what they wanted in return. I knew that no one would do something for me without wanting something back. I just didn't deserve it.

- *Fear of being intimate* — I learned that getting close to someone would inevitably bring pain because they would eventually leave. To protect myself from abandonment by someone I cared about, I tried never to care too much. When I felt myself beginning to care deeply, I would end the relationship.
- *Fear of being happy* — I often suppressed a feeling of excitement or happiness because disappointment usually followed. I believed that "what goes up, must come down."

To deal with my fears, I tried to control everything around me. Obviously, I could never successfully control my circumstances, therefore I was always terrified of being out of control. I hated it. Being in control meant surviving. I felt in control when I was slim and when I controlled my food intake. When I gained weight, I felt out of control.

It was only when I ate that I felt relief. My fear dissolved. I felt so peaceful, everything was all right — ah... I felt so safe, secure, warm and loved, like a baby feels when it is being fed. I finally felt good. I could think about anything or anyone — nothing bothered me when I was eating.

Before I began to write and talk about my fear, it consumed me. I was terrified of being abandoned and left alone. My life was driven by fear. I didn't know how to cope with all this fear; it was so painful. I couldn't stand to feel this way any longer — I had to escape.

Five

MY
ESCAPE

D*elicious, just delicious. The vanilla cream cake was so sweet, so light and so tasty. Before my next bite, I took a deep breath and exhaled all my stress. My stress was vaporizing into the air like steam from a kettle. I felt so much relief. Then, I felt strong, a strength that had not been there before. I thought about all the things I could do. I could conquer the world. I felt so powerful and so brave. I could be anybody and anything. I felt no limits, no barriers and no end to the many possibilities in life. I thought about the special man in my life and all that we could do together. I felt no negatives. I only felt wonderful. And I wondered how I ever felt otherwise. I kept eating. I was in ecstasy.*

I lived to feel pleasure, only pleasure, and never pain. Pain came up when I acknowledged "reality" *(the state of being actual or true; the state which exists objectively and in fact[1])*. Reality is experienced in the present, in the moment, in the now. And I hated the present! It was in the present that I felt alone, scared and unsafe. In the present, I was a bad person. I couldn't stand to feel more fear, shame or guilt. So, I refused to face reality and denied my painful feelings — and by doing so, denied myself access to the now, to the present.

The key to evading pain was denying reality. As long as I remained unaware of a situation, I didn't have to face my feelings about it. (If I wasn't aware that there was a lion beside me, I couldn't be afraid of it!) I was terrified of experiencing reality. I often pretended that a fact or event was not real, that it hadn't really happened. I just wouldn't acknowledge it.

I employed many strategies to avoid and ignore reality. I would get lost in my thoughts, focus on the past or the future instead of the present, get hyperactive, isolate myself and refuse to talk about it and deal with it.

I would think all the time. Have you ever tried to think and feel at the same time? It's not easy. I would think and think and think, and then

---

[1]Reader's Digest, *Reader's Digest Illustrated Encyclopedic Dictionary*, (Pleasantville, New York: The Reader's Digest Association, Inc., 1987), p 1400.

think some more. When my mind was filled with thoughts, even the most painful emotion couldn't penetrate. My thoughts shielded me from my emotions. From the moment I woke up in the morning to the moment I went to sleep, my mind was filled with thoughts. I conjured up past experiences that made me feel loved and safe, preferring to dwell on those experiences instead of experiencing new ones. I relived excerpts of my past over and over again.

When I was at work, my body was present but my mind was off somewhere else, like planning my evening. I'd tell myself: "When I get home, I'm going to kick off my shoes, make a nice dinner, relax and watch television. It'll be so relaxing. I'll be happy then." When I did get home, I might take off my shoes, but then I'd pace. I'd think about what I was going to do. I certainly wouldn't sit on the couch and relax. That would be such a waste of time. Then, I'd think about what I was going to do the next night. The next night would come, and I would think about what I would do the following weekend. I was sure that I would enjoy myself — next time. There was always tomorrow.

I was the world's greatest worrier. I worried about what had already happened and what could happen. I worried about what happened yesterday, last week and last year. I worried about what could happen next week, next month or next year. Many of my sentences began with: What if... What if they took my words the wrong way? What if they didn't think I was slim enough? What if I can't pay the rent? What if he meets someone else? What if I can't do the job? I could come up with the wildest what if's. (I'm still amazed at my imaginative ability). I worried for hours.

When I hit a mind block with "what ifs", I would resort to "if only." I'd think: "If only I hadn't said that, he would still be with me"; or "If only I hadn't driven down that street, I wouldn't have had that accident"; or "If only I hadn't told him how I felt, he would still like me"; or "If only I was skinny, everything would be great!" I wanted so badly to change events in the hopes that it would make the present better. I dwelled on what might have been. I once heard a friend say: "Today is the tomorrow you worried about yesterday." Bull's eye.

It was only talking about a situation, putting it into words, that made it real. Only then would it need to be dealt with. I believed that not talking about an issue or event would make it disappear entirely. Have you ever been in a situation when something obvious has happened, and nobody says anything? Sometimes I think that if a bomb had gone off next to me, I could convince myself it hadn't happened, just by refusing to verbally acknowledge it. That would allow me to continue about my business. (Perhaps an exaggeration, but only a slight one.)

I often suppressed comments because I didn't want to raise a painful issue or ruin a perfectly enjoyable evening. After time had passed, it would be yesterday's news anyway. I figured that yesterday was over, so why bring it up? So I didn't. But avoiding it, denying it and ignoring it didn't make it go away. It remained very much there, but unresolved.

I made myself very busy. I did and did and did. I read, went jogging, cleaned the house, played my guitar, and did whatever else I could think of doing. But, at night, I would lie in bed feeling like I had missed the day. In fact, I had. I hadn't stopped to "smell the roses." When someone called me to see how I was doing, I would always say: "I'm busy, very busy." I was! I had to stay one step ahead of my feelings.

I denied myself access to distressing feelings by "swallowing" them. When a painful emotion arose, I would respond instantly by suppressing it. I wouldn't let myself have a chance to feel it. I'd quickly replace the feeling with something pleasurable. I couldn't let anything bother me. I could swallow my fear, shame or guilt, anytime. All I had to do was eat. In fact, I got so good at it, that I swallowed feelings even before I realized I had them. I had to have complete control of my feelings. I escaped reality into a world of pleasure. I escaped to wherever I wanted to go and felt whatever pleasure I desired. My adventure began. I employed many strategies to do this: eating, fantasizing, watching television, emotionally replacing people and things, and isolating myself.

When I was eating, I felt connected. I felt connected to everything, everyone and the entire world around me. I felt wonderful, lovable and completely serene. I felt in touch with my feelings, without the pain. Before each binge, I'd feel desperate, overwhelmed. I'd exclaim: "Oh God, I can't stand it! Get me away from here! I need food!" Food would relieve my pain on contact. Food was my rescuer. It seemed almost human. When I needed relief, I had to binge.

I also had a very rich fantasy life! My fantasies were make-believe, mental illusions, beautiful dreams. When I fantasized, I climbed out of reality and into a beautiful, soft, warm and luxurious bubble, within my head. I lived in my own world, like Alice in Wonderland. I didn't acknowledge anything outside my fantasy world. Inside, I felt safe from hurt, pain and all negativity. No one could touch me.

In my illusory world I could be anything, go anywhere and do everything I wanted. I was in complete control as the director, producer and editor of my fantasies. I'd fantasize about excitement and stimulation. I'd fantasize about how much I loved my boyfriend, how breathtakingly beautiful I looked when I walked into the bar and all the men stared in awe, how gracefully I danced on the ballet stage and how passionately in love I felt when my knight in shining armour whisked me off into the sunset. I fantasized about what could happen to me that evening, week or weekend. My fantasies consisted of romantic people who loved and approved of me, places that were beautiful, warm, and things that enabled me to enjoy my beautiful life.

I stayed safe in my home as much as I could and watched television, mostly soap operas. Soap operas were my feeling window to the world. I could experience so many emotions just by watching television. I laughed, cried, felt excited and felt invigorated when I watched the soaps. The characters were very real to me — I knew them intimately. I felt everything I wanted to feel from the real world, without the risk. I could travel to places with my feelings that I'd never dare to in real life, all in the safety of my own home.

I couldn't stand to feel the pain of losing someone. I would try to replace any loss of relationship right away, so I always had a boyfriend. When I was seven, my parents separated and my mother moved away. I immediately replaced my mother with a family friend who, after my mother's departure, lived with us. I already knew her and felt loved by and safe with her. I didn't cry when my mother left — I only looked forward to my life, including the newest addition to our family. By age seven, I had already mastered the art of denial!

Not only did I replace people, but also material things. I didn't replace material things casually, as though they were luxury items. I couldn't bear their absence. I would make sure that I had more than one of whatever was special to me. I was afraid that once an item was gone, it would be gone forever and I'd have to live without it. I never wanted to live without — I'd panic at the thought. I had shoes, earrings, clothes, and make-up to last me twenty years. I needed, not wanted, to have a cushion of those material things, to be ready for — doomsday! I wore and used few of them, they often remained in the closet, jewelry box or storage, so they would always be there. I never felt shameful or guilty about having these items. I felt safe because I had them. One day, I bought a suit I loved only to store it in the closet; I would not wear it. I couldn't figure out why, I had been wanting it for days before I actually bought it. Finally I realized that if I don't wear it, it will be out of style! Initially, I had difficulty wearing it, I was so scared to damage it, but finally I enjoyed it very much. (It never did get damaged or lost.)

By isolating myself, I didn't risk exposure to pain. Being alone was safe. Also, I could finally relax and be myself. I could never relax with other people. I needed to be by myself, away from people, away from having to be someone acceptable. I could really "let go" when I was alone. Unfortunately, when I was isolated, I was lonely, but not for long. I had my food. I finally "let go," and relaxed fully, and ate.

I was searching for something, but I didn't know what. Nothing brought long-term relief — not food, not fantasies, not anything. I tried to keep my head above water to survive this horribly painful life. I vowed to live in my head, in my thoughts and fantasies, far from my heart.

Six

MY HEAD
AND HEART

I *was in a restaurant, about to eat lunch, and I couldn't decide what to order. One part of me wanted the lasagna. Another part said, like a parent disciplining a child: "Forget it, it's too fattening." Almost everything was too fattening. I looked for a dish that was more acceptable. A buffet that included salad, meat and pasta seemed like a good alternative. I decided to order the buffet and just have the salad. However, one part of me wanted to try just a little bit of the pasta ("just a teeny bit, I promise"). The other part prevailed: "No way, the pasta is off limits! Have the salad."*

That lunch took place at the beginning of my recovery. It was the first time that I really became aware of the kind of exchange that took place in my head all the time. It seemed as though my thoughts were having a dispute and I was caught helplessly in the middle. I felt like the defendant waiting for the jury to reach a verdict. I soon realized that my thoughts engaged in such a heated debate before every meal, in fact, before everything I wanted to do. Actually, by this point in my life, the discussion was more like an out-and-out battle.

I decided to pay very close attention to what was going on with my thoughts. Over time, I came to recognize that my thoughts originated from two places, and were akin to a prosecution and a defence. I called my thoughts entities because they had almost human qualities. One part of me was the disciplinarian — the prosecution. I couldn't cross her, or else! She was ready to pounce the minute I slipped. She controlled my life. The other part was a free spirit — the defence. She was the one who got prosecuted and pounced on, the one who longed to do as she wanted. She challenged the disciplinarian. Then, there was a third part — me — the helpless bystander caught in the middle. Each time my thoughts had it out, I would await the verdict, and then act on it.

The more I observed my thoughts, the more I understood them. Here's what I found. The three entities within me were my "Head," "Heart" and "Me," and each existed independently. (Although I became aware of these entities during my recovery, they still exist within me, but today they coexist much more peacefully.) I learned to see where my thoughts came from because each entity had its own distinct characteristics.

My Head is like a parent within me, the one who pounces on me. My Head forms thoughts based on what I see, hear, smell, touch and taste, and then stores these thoughts in my memory. This memory includes what I've learned, primarily from home, through parents, brothers and sisters, and from school, through teachers, peers and friends. My Head holds my values, morals, judgments, prejudices, punishments and rewards. My Head responds with thoughts about right and wrong, good and bad, acceptable and inappropriate. She watches and directs me, ensuring that my Heart behaves. Parents, teachers and authority figures often relate to the world in the same way that my Head relates to me.

My Heart is my spirit and soul — who I am at my very core. My Heart is love. At the centre of my being, it is completely aware of my true needs and wants. My Heart is what drives my energy in motion ("e-motion"). My Heart lives to feel and to love. From my Heart comes my energy, desire, motivation, purpose, destiny, drive, intuition, wisdom and love. My Heart is the kid in me. My Heart was born into this life, ready to love, live, feel, need, see, cry, do, try, and most of all, be myself.

My Head only thinks about who I am. I don't have to go looking for my desires, my feelings or my drives, they're right there in my Heart. When I'm motivated by my Heart, I'm never too tired to do anything. I'm never too tired to play tennis, but I'm always too tired to write that letter I should write. Have you ever heard the saying "her heart just wasn't in it"? My Heart isn't in anything that comes only from my Head.

My Heart has both masculine and feminine characteristics. The active, masculine side is a thinking, more aggressive side, and the other, feminine side, is a more feeling, nurturing side. The active, less emotional part of my Heart expresses assertiveness, aggressiveness, competitiveness and intellect. It expresses reason, ideas, and logic, both clearly and succinctly. This part of me learns, wonders, tries, risks, explores and is curious. My interest in climbing trees and participating in business come from this part of my Heart.

The feminine, nurturing, more feeling side of my Heart protects and loves. This side allows me to express myself with creativity, affection, joy, love and compassion. As well, I can offer care, trust, acceptance, understanding and support. This part of my Heart believes that it's okay to be sad, angry or happy. It feeds me when I'm hungry, covers me with a blanket when I'm cold, allows me to cry when I'm sad and protects me from danger. My desire to be creative through guitar/sewing and to fall in love came from this part of my Heart. Both sides complement each other to form a whole loving Heart.

The third entity, Me, is usually the helpless bystander in the midst of the battle between my Head and Heart, and the part that carries out the winning verdict. I often felt as though I had no control over what I did or didn't do. I often found myself in the most uncomfortable places with people I didn't want to be with. I had just helplessly acted, without conscious awareness. I felt like I had no say in the matter. I had been letting my Head make most of the decisions. I would get so upset when my boyfriend made a decision without involving me. Now I knew why. A part of me was making decisions without involving me. And I was miserable.

I had been making dozens of choices a day, without realizing how I arrived at them. My Head and Heart related to each other as two powerful opponents in battle. My Head thought — only. My Head responded to a situation with thoughts about what I should do. I acted only after I had thought something through. My Head tried to make the right choice or, the best decision for everyone concerned. The right choices always seemed to be what other people thought I should do. My Head listened to everyone but my Heart.

My Head's voice was dominant. She was like an authoritative parent who controlled and restricted me in every way. My Head watched every move my Heart made. My Head accepted or rejected my Heart's desires. My Head parented me as I had been by my real-life parents. My Head disciplined me and gave me rewards and punishments similar to those I had received while growing up. My Head rejected and punished my Heart with many hurtful and denigrating thoughts. My Head shamed me, made me feel guilt, fear and doubt. When I wanted pasta, my Head pounced: "Forget it, you don't need to gain any more weight than you already have. (shame)" She pounced: "If you eat the pasta, you'll just worry about the weight you probably gained from it. (fear)" She pounced: "You won't have just a little bit of the pasta. (doubt)" She finished her pouncing by limiting me: "You can only have the salad."

When my Head was in ascendance, I experienced the following feelings: the need to control and protect; a need for safety; a longing for the approval and acceptance of others; shame; a need for perfection; fear; doubt; judgment; comparison; guilt; punishment; reward; worry and projection; denial; a reaction to habit; mistrust; dishonesty; role playing; invalidation of feelings; inability to handle emotion; jealousy, envy; inability to be intimate; and difficulty in having fun.

The other voice, barely heard, was from my Heart. My Heart wanted to eat the pasta and order whatever she wanted from the menu.

On the day I described above, at first my Head seemed to win the battle over lunch, but not for long. I did have the salad from the buffet. But then I went for seconds. I put a little pasta beside my salad, just to have a taste. I went up a third time and filled my plate with lasagna, pizza and meatballs. On the fourth plate, I had chocolate pudding, cheesecake and a brownie. The fifth was laden with a slice of lemon meringue pie, two butter tarts and more pudding. I had more lasagna on the last plate.

In the end, my Heart won out. It won every time I binged. My Heart just wanted to enjoy some, not huge amounts, of food, tasty food. By starving, depriving myself of food, especially delicious food, to compensate, I ate and ate and ate. I wanted the pasta but my Head wouldn't let me have it. When I finally let myself have "just a little," the leash was loosened, just enough for my Heart to escape. I binged. I had been deprived for too long. I needed pleasure. I overdosed. I couldn't seem to help it.

I binged on food when what I was really hungering for was love from my Heart, my nurturing side. My Head ensured that I had little contact with my Heart. My Head was so cruel to me. My Head deprived me. My Heart wanted, needed and desired to fill me up.

Before I began my recovery, I did not acknowledge "Me." I certainly did not stop to choose whether I wanted to binge. I just did it. I didn't see a choice. I (the Me) acted on the thoughts of my Head most of the time. I didn't realize that I could have chosen to eat some of the pasta, and it wouldn't have hurt me. To me, the choice as all or nothing, binge or starve — no in-between.

In choosing to follow my Head for so many years, I sacrificed the natural path of my Heart. I ignored its feelings and desires. My Head saw all the hurt I had experienced, all the shame that I received, and all the anger and pain I had caused others as truly bad. My Head wanted no part of me. My Heart was me. My Head split away from my Heart, from Me. I began to live as a divided/split person. I never felt like I belonged to anything. I didn't even belong to myself.

Living this way was like living between three people, each with opposing views on what was right. My entities fought each other constantly. They did anything but work together toward a common goal. My Head related to the world only from her side, fear. My Head tried to make me shine, gain love and acceptance. My Head could never shine like the sun — my Heart already was.

At birth, I was equipped with all the tools necessary for me to fully participate in the world — I was whole. Had I based my choices on and then acted on the energy from my Heart, I would have been whole. From the time I was born, to the miracle of my recovery, I travelled full circle. I went from being a whole person to a divided person and back to being a whole person again.

As if I were turning the handle on a kaleidoscope, my perception of myself was slowly beginning to change. I had been so sure that I was who I thought I was. I was progressing. Although I still felt fearful, I felt energized. I was growing closer to myself.

Seven

HOW I
LEARNED MY
THOUGHTS

pon waking, I immediately started berating myself. "Oh God, why did you have to eat the whole bag of crackers last night?" I had eaten too much again and I felt awful. Another failure. I scolded myself: "Damn! I can't believe you did that. Whose side are you on anyway? Well, you can't eat until three o'clock this afternoon. That'll fix it. You must lose weight! At least the weight you gained from all those crackers." In the shower, thoughts poured into my mind. What I would do at work, whether to resolve the dispute with my co-worker, and what to wear to cover the weight I'd gained. I couldn't stop this flood of thoughts. I put my hands over my ears and shook my head, trying to keep my mind from exploding.

I knew that my thoughts came from my Head, but how did they get in there? Where did they come from? How did I draw certain conclusions? Why did I feel so compelled to lose weight? Why did I get so crazy when I saw certain people? Why did I panic when I came into contact with certain things? Why did I feel so sad when I heard a song on the radio? Why did I feel so safe when I smelled a familiar scent? Was it possible that I was reacting to something that had happened in the past? The answer, I was to discover, was an irrevocable yes!

I used to laugh when I'd see a psychiatrist and a client in therapy on a television show. The psychiatrist would be sure to ask about the client's childhood. What did that have to do with anything, I recall wondering. Why do psychiatrists always ask about it? Now, I know that my childhood had everything to do with everything.

I learned all of my thoughts. I learned my thoughts from my experiences.

I knew which thoughts came from my Head and which from my Heart. However, paying attention to them was full-time work! There were millions of them and they played against the screen of my mind all the time. If at first, I didn't understand the meaning of a certain thought, I always got a second chance. I had many of the same thoughts over and over again. I became aware that my responses followed a sequence — one I could anticipate.

Certain people, places and things caused me to respond in certain ways. When I was in contact with food, I felt guilty for wanting it, afraid that I would gain weight from it and ashamed for binging on it. I responded to food very emotionally. It had long ago lost its physical significance. I knew that something, other than what was present in the now, was triggering me to respond. I responded to food the same way, every time.

This is the sequence I followed: (1) contact a stimulus; (2) experience a stimulus; (3) respond to this experience emotionally and physically and; (4) form a conclusion, i.e., a "message" or a "thought" based on this.

A "stimulus" is something that causes a response. I respond when I contact something, such as a person, place, or thing, including the physical senses of sight (view), sound (music), taste (food), touch (hugs), smell (cologne).

From the moment I entered the world, I experienced life and I've been affected by everything that I've ever experienced. I have responded to every "experience." An experience is what happens to me and the lessons I learn when I contact a stimulus. I experienced weight gain when I ate too much food. I experienced criticism for having gained weight. I attached the criticism to food. I blamed food for it.

A "response" is a reaction to an experience. I "responded" to every experience in two ways, with my Head and my Heart — by "feeling" (emotional) and by "doing" (physical). I ate too much food (stimulus), gained weight and heard criticism (experience). I responded to my experience by feeling terrified (response — feeling) and then, feeling the pain of rejection and fearing abandonment, I went on a diet (response — doing).

A "message" is a collection of specific thoughts from the Head. I formed a message, a conclusion from my experiences. I accepted a message as true and stored it into memory. Ah ha! This was the key! This is where my "thoughts" came from! I had heard the message that if I wasn't thin, people would criticize and reject me. Therefore, I must lose weight. As though that message played over a loud speaker, I heard it loud and clear. I finally saw a thought, a message, for what it was!

Throughout my life, I had gotten the message! Whether or not someone spoke to me, I would form a conclusion about them, me and the experience. When someone turned up their nose at me, I got the message that they thought I was disgusting. I was very perceptive.

Here's how it worked when it came to food. This was the sequence: Stimulus—> Experience—> Response (feel/do) —> Message (thought). Once I formed a message, I attached the message to the stimulus. I had attached criticism to food. I would respond to a message, not an experience. Once I had experienced criticism after having gained weight, I thought that I would always be criticized if I gained weight. So, I responded by always dieting. After I had learned this message, I never related to food normally again. Food represented pain, weight gain, criticism and rejection. I began to resent food.

When I contacted a "stimulus" that had a message attached to it, I would: Think (message) -> Feel (emotional response) -> Do (action response)

Once I recorded my message, I responded to it every time I contacted the same or a similar stimulus. It was as though the message was carved in stone, as though it were absolute truth and reality. My thoughts hypnotized me. They captured my full attention. Someone could press any stimulus button and I would react according to its message. I lived according to my thoughts. If I thought something would be enjoyable, I would feel good. If I thought I wouldn't like to do something, I would feel negatively about it. I tried to stay away from all stimuli that had painful messages attached to it. I would leave a restaurant if I saw a person I didn't want to talk to. I wouldn't go to a party if my boyfriend didn't want me to go. I wouldn't order the food I really wanted because it might make me fat.

I felt very uncomfortable around food and tried to stay far away from it. It had the most powerful message attached to it. It could make me gain weight and be rejected. I starved myself to dizziness. I purged, even though it was extremely painful. I didn't care how hungry, tired or dizzy I felt. All the side-effects in the world would not stop me: I had to be skinny. There was no debate. I acted, whether rationally or not, on all my messages, without question. My messages were incredibly powerful!

I learned most of my messages when I was young and unable to understand why an experience had occurred. Had I been able to understand what was really going on, I might have created different messages. When a toy is removed from a child and the child wants to continue playing with it, the child may cry, not understanding why it was removed. When toys were removed from me, I didn't know why. I didn't understand what caused things to come, go, hurt, or feel bad; I simply experienced those situations and formed my own conclusions, messages.

Once a messages had formed, it went into my memory and I reacted to it. I remembered very few of the experiences that taught me these messages. I might have been five years old when I learned a message and yet I would respond to it and have the very same feeling at 25.

My Head tried to protect, control, dominate my life. She tried to ensure that I would never have to hurt again. Since my Head had split off and become emotionally disconnected from the painful messages in my Heart, my Heart was left lifeless and breathless.

I had been responding to my old messages, instead of to the reality of the situation. The thoughts that raced through my head every morning when I awoke were the result of 25 years of learning. Some thoughts were new and some were two years old. I looked back to my past to discover where my messages originated. I came to realize that I had some very basic messages that had affected my life profoundly. I finally learned what had made me feel so sad, afraid, guilty and shameful.

Eight

MY BASIC
MESSAGES

One night, I was lying in bed, crying loudly. I looked up and saw my father. Then came the spanking. I was five at the time. I was filled with terror. I was certain no one cared about me. All I wanted was to be held, to feel safe. But now I felt worse — I just wanted to die. I had gotten what I deserved. I was alone with my pain and fear. I had no doubt that I would always be alone. I rolled over in bed, pressed my face down hard on my mattress, and put my pillow over my head. I whimpered. I was too scared to sob. I was scared to be scared. I was scared and alone.

Growing up, I always felt alone, even though our house was full of people. I wanted so much to be included, to be a part of the activity of life, but I felt that I'd never be a part of anything. My interpretation of my experiences taught me that I was alone, and would be alone forever. I carried with me the most basic, most devastating message to prove it.

Once I understood how I had learned my messages, I began to look at my experiences. At first, I had a hard time, I drew blanks. I could barely remember anything before the age of five. But by making a concerted and conscious effort, it wasn't long before I remembered bits and pieces. Every time I felt shame, guilt, fear or pain, I would ask myself when I had felt the same thing in the past. Often, I could recall a situation from my childhood in which those feelings resonated. That's how I remembered most of my experiences — I felt my way back to my childhood. I didn't regain total memory, but I did start to recall my feelings. I gained an incredible appreciation for how profound an impact they had had on me. I developed tremendous compassion for myself.

I absorbed messages from experiences at home with my family, school, friends and their homes, places I socialized, books and media, the workplace with coworkers, and from the public. However, none of my messages were more potent than the ones I learned in the first five years of my life. The messages learned then were the messages I responded to as true, until my recovery. Those messages were my *basic messages*. I was living my life according to the information they contained. My messages were my interpretation of reality, not necessarily what actually happened.

No two people affected me more than my parents. They were my role models. I learned messages by how they related to me, to each other, and to society. I don't blame my parents or anyone else in any way for my experiences or my messages. Initially, when I began my recovery, I wanted to make someone responsible for my pain. I felt cheated from happiness. I was angry. Soon afterward, I realized that no one was to blame, not even me. I would have preferred to have completed this book without having to mention my parents. This book is about me, not them. However, I believe it would be remiss not to mention how I perceived my most significant influence, and how their actions affected me.[1]

One day I was reading a psychology text and found myself staring at a chart in amazement. It was Erik Erikson's Psychosocial Stages of Development. This chart described so perfectly the route of growth I had taken. Unfortunately, the terms that so accurately described my path were on the right side of the word "versus" (see below). In my development, I took the road of mistrust, doubt, guilt, inferiority, confusion and isolation. Given this, the fact that my outcomes were not favourable should come as no surprise.

I'm very happy to share the following information. It helped me gain a much clearer picture of how I had drawn many of my conclusions and incorporated many messages. It helped me understand the stage I was in when I learned certain messages that I responded to later. Broken down, the term "psychosocial stage of development" means: " psycho" — *mental view of oneself,* "social" — *in relation to others;* "stage" — *over a period of time;* "development" — *relating to growth.*

Erikson's stages of psychosocial development illustrate that problems relating to other people change with age. He defines eight major life stages in terms of the psychosocial problems, or crises, that must be resolved in each. (Chart below, After Erikson, 1963)[2]

---

[1] I don't believe that anyone intentionally set out to hurt me. Unfortunately, much hurt is passed around in this world, but I don't believe for a moment that anyone likes to give or receive it. I don't believe there is a perfect parent or a perfect person. I'm grateful for the many wonderful experiences I did have with my family.

[2] Rita L. Atkinson, Richard C. Atkinson, Edward E. Smith, Daryl J. Bem, *Introduction to Psychology*, Tenth Edition, (Orlando, Florida: Harcourt Brace Javanovich, 1990), p 108.

STAGES	PSYCHOLOGICAL CRISES	FAVOURABLE OUTCOME
1. First year of life	Trust versus mistrust	Trust and optimism
2. Second year	Autonomy versus doubt	Sense of self-control and adequacy
3. Third through sixth year	Initiative versus guilt	Purpose and direction Ability to initiate one's own activities
4. Sixth year to adolescence	Industry versus inferiority	Competence in intellectual, social, and physical skills
5. Adolescence	Identity versus confusion	An integrated image of oneself as a unique person
6. Early adulthood	Intimacy versus isolation	Ability to form close and lasting relationships; to make career commitments
7. Middle adulthood	Generativity versus self-absorption	Concern for family, society, and future generations
8. The aging years	Integrity versus despair	A sense of fulfilment and satisfaction with one's life; willingness to face death

STAGE ONE: Trust versus Mistrust

Trust is having faith and optimism. This is the stage in which I learned my messages of fear and mistrust. My experiences during the first 23 days of my life shaped the way I related to myself, to others, and to the world, throughout my life. When I was born, my birth mother was 16 years old and in grade 11. She delivered twins at the Toronto General Hospital in Ontario, Canada. My twin sister and I were put up for adoption and adopted into the same family. (For that I am very grateful.) After we were born, we remained in the hospital for 13 days. I remained for an additional 10 days. For the first 23 days my life, I was alone — without my mother. My twin sister, with whom I had shared a safe haven for nine months, was also gone.

During those 23 days, I experienced being abandoned by my biological mother. Birth pulled me from the warm, safe haven of the womb into a cold, loud world. I was not greeted or hugged by my biological mother. I lived in an incubator, all alone. I was fed according to the clock, not according to my need. That experience has had devasting effects on me. During my first 23 days, I was more vulnerable than I would ever be again. From that experience, I learned four of my most basic and potent messages:

1. I will die if I am abandoned.
2. I can never trust that someone will be there for me.
3. I am shameful and unlovable.
4. My needs and wants are bad.

Message 1: I will die if I am abandoned (fear).

I concluded that I could never survive abandonment. At this age, I was helpless and completely dependent on others for my survival. I couldn't survive without being fed and changed by the nurses, and I couldn't survive without my parents to take care of me. My fears of not surviving abandonment were valid. (Later, every time I detected the possibility of abandonment, I panicked as though I were being abandoned as I had been at birth).

Throughout my life, I would wake up in the middle of the night, in the morning, or after a nap and feel an overwhelming, sickening pain — terrified and alone. I didn't want to be in this cold cruel world. For 25 years, I responded to everyone and everything around me with the fear and expectation that I'd be abandoned once again. *All of my fears were based on this message.*

Message 2: Never trust anyone (lack of faith).

I didn't trust anyone to be there for me. No one was there for me when I was born, when I was in the most need. I wasn't fed when I was hungry, but according to the clock. I wasn't welcomed into this world by my biological mother I never felt truly welcome anywhere. I learned never to depend on anyone to be there for me. I hated to depend or be dependent on anyone. I tried to never allow myself to be vulnerable. I held back from being open or honest with anyone in order to lessen my vulnerability.

I didn't allow myself to hope. The moment I felt hopeful about something, it would be followed by a dull feeling of impending doom. Things were always too good to be true. I knew that somehow, everything would be ruined. If it didn't get ruined by outside circumstance, I would ruin it. I couldn't stand to be surprised by bad fate.

I had no faith in God. I had no faith in anything good or positive. Faith requires trust. I didn't trust that things would work out for the best. How could my experience after my birth have been for the best? I had been warm and safe in the womb. Suddenly, to my surprise, all that changed and I lost all of that safety. After my birth, I never felt safe. I wouldn't "let go" of my control and trust that fate would prevail. I had no choice but to be "out of control" when I was born, but I could try to compensate for that afterwards.

My mission in life was to regain the feeling of being in the womb, to be warm, fed and safe. I fed myself and I felt very safe when I did. Forget trusting that "things always have a way of working out." Forget fate. I swore I would never be vulnerable again!

Message 3: I am shameful and unlovable.

I concluded that I was shameful because no one had been there for me when I was born, so I must be a terribly unlovable person. If I had been a good person, then my biological mother wouldn't have abandoned me. All of my feelings of shame were based on this message. I learned that I'm alone in this world, because I'm not lovable. When my father spanked me instead of hugging me when I cried, I resonated with the pain I had experienced after my birth. Obviously, I wasn't worthy of being hugged. I always felt alone. I was alone in an incubator in a room full of babies, and I was alone in a house full of people.

Message 4: My needs and wants are bad.

I learned that all of my needs and wants (my Heart) were bad. I didn't deserve to have them satisfied because I was shameful. If I wasn't bad, they would have been satisfied immediately. I would have had the love and affection of my biological mother and she would have fed me immediately when I was hungry and changed my diaper when it needed to be. My needs and wants were not met, especially my need for love and comfort. A nurse cannot replace a mother. So after the first 23 days of my life, I didn't trust that someone would be there for me. I didn't feel safe or secure. I didn't hope for safety.

Upon release from the hospital, my twin sister and I began our life in Toronto with our adoptive parents, and a brother who was two years old at the time. The next year we moved to the east coast, and lived in New Brunswick and Nova Scotia for five years. During the first two years, we had two additions to our family. In the first year, there was an adopted brother who was three years old, and the year after that, my mother gave birth to my younger sister.

At the end of stage one, at one year old, I had chosen mistrust. I did not trust anyone or anything, not even myself. I didn't feel safe in this world.

Nine

I
DOUBTED
MYSELF

STAGE TWO: Autonomy versus Doubt
(Age 2)

"**N**o!...Don't... Stop! What have you done now? Stop your crying. Go to your room." I put my hands over my ears. I couldn't stand it anymore. I wished they would just stop saying those things to me. I can't do anything right! Either they yell at me or take my toys away. I can't have any fun anymore. Everything I try, I do wrong. I'm being yelled at from all directions. I don't know where to turn. Why am I so bad? Why do I cause all this yelling? Will I ever be able to do anything right?

Many parents know this stage as "the terrible twos." At first, I thought: "Wow, I have some control over myself! I can walk! I'm no longer stuck." I was no longer totally dependent and helpless. I had stepped into the stage of exploration.

Erik Erikson describes "autonomy" as: *the act of being independent and self-contained. A person can begin to build a relationship with one's self which includes self-love, self-care, self-trust.* I didn't come to the conclusion that I was autonomous. If I had, it would have meant acknowledging that I was separate from my parents and capable of functioning independently of them. I would have built a relationship with myself that included self-love, self-care, self-trust. However, I hated who I was, didn't take care of myself and never ever trusted myself. Not only didn't I have a relationship with myself, but it was as though I was a perfect stranger, who felt only distaste and disgust for me. The last thing I wanted to do was begin a relationship with me.

I was in my second year of life, and for the first time I could explore and experience my world. I could finally do things instead of just stay in a crib. I was out of my crib and in the real world, filled with excitement. I had so much to learn, so much to do. I was curious about everything. I tried to do many different things, once I had learned to crawl and then walk. I tried to put blocks together, I played with my brothers and sisters, and I began to speak. I tested my own potentials and limits. It was in this stage that I learned how shameful I was.

As I began my exploration of the world, I was extremely vulnerable. This was my first attempt and my most critical and influential experience of being me. I needed someone to guide me, lovingly and gently, through this stage. I needed my parents' feedback as a sounding board.

I learned about who I was by how they responded to me and my actions. They were like a mirror. I looked to see their reaction every time I did something. They revealed their acceptance or rejection through their facial expressions, tone of voice and actions. If they smiled, I was good. If they yelled and spanked me, I was bad. If their reaction was positive, I felt accepted and safe. If their reaction was negative, I felt rejected and scared of being abandoned. Throughout my life, I would interpret people's reactions in a similar way.

I didn't know then that I was separate from my behaviour. I hadn't learned that I was separate from my parents and their response to me. When I did something wrong and was told: "You dummy, that's not how you do it"; or "How stupid can you be?" and I concluded that there was something wrong with me, not my behaviour. I learned messages of self-doubt, self-disgust and self-hate during this stage. I learned messages of shame (see Chapter 3) during this stage. I experienced great frustration. I was limited and punished for my self-expression.

I learned three basic messages in this stage:

1. I doubt I can do it.
2. I can't be separated from my parents and survive.
3. I can't deal with my feelings.

Message 1: I doubt I can do it.

I got their message. I knew what they meant when they told me "no," "stop," "don't," and "you dummy." In utter frustration, I gasped: "What's wrong with me?" There had to be something terribly wrong with me, since I couldn't do anything right. I felt so worthless and incapable. I just wanted to do what I wanted and be who I wanted, and I couldn't understand why I wasn't allowed to. (In chapter 22, I describe how verbal violations affected me.)

As an adult, when someone said "no" or "don't," I reacted in the same way to the same feelings of frustration and shame. I would ask: "What do you expect me to do?" Or, "How do you expect me to feel?" Or, "I can't do anything right." I felt so shameful when I couldn't do something. By doubting myself, I had given up my chance to become autonomous.

Message 2: I can' be separated from my parents and survive.

I decided that I had better stop what I was doing now before I made things even worse. So, I stopped trying, exploring, or doing anything that made them yell. Everything that I wanted made them yell and I hated it. I was really afraid that were going to abandon me. I began to behave. I learned that when I didn't behave according to what parents wanted, they yelled. I must stop doing everything that makes them yell. I became a good girl.

I felt separated from my parents when they yelled at me, and I was afraid of being separated from my parents. I didn't trust that they would be around when I returned. Instead of exploring the world around me, I worried about being abandoned. I didn't trust that all would be okay when I wasn't with my parents.

When I was bad, my parents sent me to my room, away from everyone. Being in my room, alone without my parents, I felt rejected, abandoned and terrified. I decided that I must never be bad enough to be sent to my room. In later years, I hated to travel; I couldn't stand to be away from familiar and safe environments.

Message 3: I can't deal with my feelings.

By age two, I had learned to deny my feelings! No wonder I was so good at it, after 20 years of practice. I couldn't deal with my feelings of shame, anger and hurt, I didn't have the coping mechanisms. As a young child trying to cope with my feelings, I denied them by repressing them (see Chapter 5 — "My Escape"); I identified with the person who caused me pain (see Chapter 22 — "I Developed a Boundary") and I projected (directed) my feelings onto someone or something other than the cause. (The process of projection is called "displacement." I displaced or misplaced my feelings, I did not own them.)

When I spilled the milk on the table, I blamed my brother for pushing me into it. I displaced my feelings by blaming my brother. In my adult life, I often displaced my feelings, blaming many other people for my actions. I "took out" or projected my anger toward other people, when it was my mistake. I hadn't learned how to handle my own feelings; I hadn't owned them. I didn't know how to take responsibility for them. I didn't deal with my feelings.

I felt very angry for being restricted and punished. The more I was told "no," the more I rebelled and the angrier I became. Unfortunately, my anger just got me into more trouble. I quickly learned that if I showed my anger, I would be yelled at, not praised; I would be rejected, not accepted; I would be alone, not safe; I would be abandoned, not loved. So,

I suppressed my anger. Later, during my recovery, saying no or disagreeing was a great challenge. I feared being abandoned.

At age two, I tried to be all that I could be, yet I wasn't allowed to be myself. All the "no's" and "don'ts" had confirmed that. I failed to become a great block builder. All my life, I felt like a failure. I failed to become me, an autonomous being. I walked away from stage two believing that I couldn't do anything and that failure was inevitable.

By failing, I had given in (just like I had given in to food) to higher demands. I had to obey my parents or face the consequences. The consequences were not good. I could be yelled at or punished. Either way, I felt abandoned by them. The struggle, between my parents and me, was about me trying to be me versus what they wanted me to be. I struggled to be myself; to do what I wanted to do; to express myself in exactly the way I wanted. But I always lost. I didn't have much choice. It was either conform to my parents' wishes, or be punished. Not much of a choice. In my adult life, I believe that I tested limits in an attempt to "get away with" something in an attempt to somehow win the two-year-old struggle. I could not win.

I felt so useless, weak and inferior. I was overpowered. I had to resign to a position of loss. I was defeated. I learned that I couldn't do it. I completed this stage by giving up on myself. I had become completely dependent on my parents to tell me who I was, what I could or could not do. I took away the message that because I wasn't good enough to be myself, or strong enough to win the struggle to become autonomous, I would always have to depend on others for my survival.

The groundwork had been laid for me to crave the acceptance by others, to need to be slim, to seek desperately to avoid the pain of failing myself. I had to hold onto something or someone for my survival. I doubted I could swim so other people, things and food became my life preservers. I held onto them for dear life. I was dependent on them for survival. I could not swim.

I lived the next 23 years responding to myself and others in that way. If I hadn't chosen food, I would have become addicted to something else. Giving up myself and accepting defeat, was excruciatingly painful. So, at the end of stage two, I didn't trust that people would be there for me, I didn't feel safe, and I hadn't developed my autonomy. In short, I had no sense of myself and no boundaries.

I wouldn't let myself be the person who, if left to their own desires, would get yelled at and rejected. I wouldn't let myself express, do, feel, play or experience me in any way. I shut off my natural flow so that I would never be abandoned.

Ten

I WAS
GUILTY

STAGE THREE: Initiative versus Guilt
(Age 3-5)

I *was in the back of our stationwagon playing dominos with my sister. We were five. My family was taking one of our many driving trips. My sister and I had been given two pieces of bubble gum each. We each ate one. I told my sister to save the second one just in case someone else wanted it. I went ahead and had mine and she held onto hers. When my father asked if anyone had a piece of gum, my sister said yes and passed it to him. I was so relieved and happy that I had told her to save it. Then my mother asked for a piece. I didn't have one for her. I could have died. I felt so awful and selfish. I had taken what should have been hers. I felt extremely guilty. I vowed never to do that again.*

I felt completely responsible for everyone. It was up to me to keep my family happy and save them from painful experiences. When I failed, I felt horribly guilty. In stage two, I learned doubt instead of autonomy. Doubting myself, I looked to others to tell me what to do instead of initiating activities on my own. "Initiative" is *a person's ability to initiate one's own activities, and by doing so, gaining purpose and direction.* I waited to be told what to do.

This was the time to learn how to relate to the world. I was vulnerable and impressionable at this age. My parents were my role models, my teachers, my mirror to myself and my window to the world. I watched them closely. I learned much from them — right and wrong, good and bad. I absorbed their values and morals as well as their fear, guilt and shame. I learned about sexuality from them. I learned empathy, especially how my actions affected others. I was like a little sponge soaking up what was happening around me. Most of all, I learned guilt.

Influenced by my previous messages, I learned four more basic messages:
1. I cause others their pain.
2. My natural impulses are bad.
3. Not trying is easier.
4. I must prove that I'm not guilty.

I learned my messages of guilt (see Chapter 2) during this stage. These messages strengthened my feelings of shame.

Message 1: I cause others their pain.

When other people felt pain, I believed I was the cause. As I described in Chapter 2, I felt completely responsible for rectifying a situation that had caused another person pain. I would say "I'm sorry" every day for many years. I didn't ask for or take something when I thought someone else needed it more. When I did, I felt responsible for their loss and guilt-ridden for my gain. I felt a real struggle between what I (my Heart) wanted and a feeling of guilt (Head — messages) for getting it.

Message 2: My natural desires are bad.

All of my natural (Heart) desires were bad. In stage one, I had learned that my needs and wants were bad. In this stage, I learned that my sexuality, and my desires for fun and play were bad. My desires always got me into trouble. Anytime I acted on impulse, my parents pounced on me (just like my Head pounced on my Heart.) I felt that I was selfish for having any wants. I felt selfish for taking something for my own purpose or enjoyment. I stopped asking for my wants to be satisfied. I wished I could stop wanting, but I couldn't. I thought that I was a bad person because I couldn't control my wants.

I had wanted my gum and acted on that want. I felt so selfish for having my gum, gum that my mom wanted. I had known that I should have saved it in case someone else wanted it. That was why I told my sister not to have hers. I should have saved mine too. I caused my mom to go without. I was the one who deserved to go without, not my mom.

My desires for fun and play were bad. I would hurt someone when we wrestled, I'd laugh too loudly or I'd fall and hurt myself. I got scared when I followed my own desires, someone usually got hurt. I also felt guilty for feeling sexual. I learned that sex was dirty. I believed that my sexual desires were bad, yet I sure had them. I couldn't control my drive and I felt very guilty about not being able to control it. I couldn't seem to get rid of these exciting thoughts and fantasies.[1]

---

[1]*According to a Freudian theory, "the Oedipal Complex" is experienced during this stage. My interpretation of Freud's theory is that a boy has a sexual desire for his mother and wants her as his partner. A boy competes with his father for his mother. A boy who wishes that his father would go away or die, often feels guilty for his wishes. In time, a boy learns that his desire for his mother is wrong. A boy feels guilty for it. This*

Message 3: Not trying is easier.

I spilled the milk. I spoke when I wasn't supposed to. I cried when I wasn't supposed to. I couldn't put the blocks together. I couldn't draw. I couldn't speak properly. I couldn't get along with my brothers and sisters without fighting. I was not capable of doing most of things I tried. I would hear the message that I couldn't do something right even before I tried. I knew that I would never be able to play the piano, ride a horse or sing. (If I couldn't put blocks together, how could I ride a horse?)

When I found myself stuck up a tree, I knew that it was my fault for not having listened to my parents. If I had, I wouldn't have gotten myself into that mess. Had I been smart enough, I would have never climbed so high. When I made a mistake, I knew it was because I didn't have the capacity to do it right. I'd hear: "What's wrong with you?" I knew that something must be wrong with me, I just kept making mistakes. At four years old, I didn't know that the electrical baseboard heater would burn my fingers. So I put my fingers inside and found out! When I went crying for help, the response was: "What have you done now?" I simply didn't know any better but I always felt like I should have.

I could only do so much, make so many mistakes before I threw in the towel and said: Forget it! I couldn't see the point of trying, just to be yelled at, disciplined, burned or laughed at. I stopped trying. When I took the initiative and tried to do something, I inevitably failed. So I just stopped trying.

Message 4: I must prove that I'm not guilty.

When my parents punished me, I just wanted to just crawl under a table, I felt so ashamed. A dog lowers his head and puts his tail between his legs. I would have done the same if I could have. I wanted to just disappear. (That's one of the reasons I wanted to lose weight, to disappear.)

I tried to prove that I wasn't guilty of making my parents yell by trying to be perfect at something — at anything. If I managed — let's say to put the blocks together — I might make my parents proud or happy, and then I might not be such a bad person. But I kept trying and kept failing. I didn't want to give up becoming good, but it didn't seem to matter what I did, I could never get it right. I realized that I was guilty of making my parent's yell. I could see that I was a big disappointment, so my efforts proved futile.

---

process usually takes about two years to work out, if a person works it out. I believe that the reverse is true for girls and their fathers. (I have often wondered if having an affair is an attempt at capturing the unavailable parent? Who knows? I don't. However, I have wanted an unavailable man and have felt very guilty for it.)

My messages (Head) said that everything natural about me (Heart) was wrong and bad. At the same time, I felt an inner drive (from my Heart) to satisfy my natural drives. The result was confusion. I didn't know which to choose — the desires of my Heart or the thoughts of my Head. So I struggled. Choosing the desires of my Heart threatened abandonment, so I chose my Head. From this point onward, I listened to and responded to the messages from my Head and ignored my Heart. I gave up myself. This is where my addiction began.

In my first five years, I learned the basic messages that would govern my life: *I will die if I am abandoned. I can never trust anyone. I am shameful and unlovable. My needs and wants are bad. I doubt I can do it. I won't survive if I am separated from my parents. I can't deal with my feelings. I cause others their pain. My natural desires are bad. Not trying is easier. I must prove that I'm not guilty.* I responded to all of those messages until my recovery. So many of the decisions I would make in my life were based on those messages.

Eleven

I FELT
INFERIOR

STAGE FOUR: Industry versus Inferiority
(Age 6-12)

'd watch in awe while my classmate performed in a play. He was very good. I'd watch another jump on the trampoline in gymnastics class. She was very good. And I was not good at anything. I was so shy. I didn't get accepted into the drama class. I didn't get straight A's. I didn't make the spelling team. I didn't have what it took. I couldn't do anything right. I didn't feel I belonged. I wished that I could be like my classmates — talented, smart and confident. But I couldn't. I was incompetent and inferior. And I knew it. I felt cheated. I wondered why I didn't have talents like theirs. What had I done? I hated being me.

From this point on, I didn't learn any new messages — I just applied the ones I already had. For the first time, I was in regular contact with other kids, parents and authority figures. I was exposed to the world outside my home. I experienced many changes during this stage. I began school, moved to four different homes, had my first serious accident, experienced my parent's divorce, experienced my first romance and went to summer camp. Through all this, I used my basic messages to help me cope.

"Industry" is *when a person gains competence in intellectual, social and physical skills.* "Competence" is *the state of being capable or competent.* To acquire competence, you have to try before you can succeed. Instead, I responded to the ingrained message: "I doubt I can do it." This stopped me from trying most things. To do well in school, I had to study, but I didn't. So when I did poorly, I could blame it on that.

There were times, however few, when I did try. I'd make a quick attempt and if I couldn't do it, I'd quit immediately and never try the same thing again. I didn't realize that most people worked very hard to achieve success.

I began this stage without the necessary tools (skill, knowledge, drive and motivation) to acquire competence. My messages told me that I was not capable of acquiring these tools. I didn't have positive messages to support messages such as: "I can do it, I am lovable, I am smart, I don't have to do it perfectly and I will not be abandoned."

Now that I was spending more time outside my home, people other than my family were exposed to my shame. Teachers at school knew how dumb I was. My report cards proved it. My teachers would fill in the comment section, beside the grade for each subject, with such remarks as: "Sheila is a student who lacks concentration and needs more motivation." My low grades confirmed their observations. Throughout my school years, I believed all my teachers knew how shameful I was.

When I did take the initiative and tried something in public, I felt horribly exposed for the incapable person I was. I usually failed. Then, not only did my family know how bad I was, the whole world knew. I felt almost naked when I was up on stage performing or speaking in the public eye. So, I withdrew from the public. I didn't enter contests. I couldn't stand for other people to see how bad I was.

I felt unworthy before other parents as well as my own. My friends' parents called me shy, and I was — excruciatingly so. I felt so horrible about myself that I would blush at the slightest gesture that I felt revealed my inadequacies. My parents' friends commented on how adorable this shyness was. If they knew how agonizing being shy really was, they wouldn't have said it was an adorable quality. It was a painful complex and I hated it. I so wished I could be outgoing like so many of my friends, but I couldn't.

I began school at the kindergarten level in Mahone Bay, Nova Scotia. My kindergarten class was more like grade one. Instead of drawing and playing, we learned to read and write. I envied kids who went to kindergarten and got to play. I had been at home with my mom for the previous five years — she had stayed at home with all of us before we began school. As long as she was around, I didn't have to fear that I would be separated from her. I knew I wouldn't survive if I was.

School was the last place I wanted to be. It was a frightening experience. My teacher was an older lady who was very strict. I have no pleasant memories of that classroom. However, now my fear seemed very real. I was being forced to go to a place where no one joked or played. I spent all day in that stressful environment. My fun was over.

One day, the principal came into the classroom with one of our classmates. They stood before us beside the teacher's desk. With a stern look on her face, the teacher said: "This boy has been bad and now he's going to get the strap. This is what each of you will get if you are bad!" The principal gave the boy the strap in front of our class. The boy screamed and cried. They had humiliated him and scared the rest of us to death. I learned that if I was bad I would get the strap and be humiliated in front of everyone. I became a very good (and very terrified) girl after that experience. School was not fun and definitely not safe. (I felt the same way about school throughout the rest of my school years.)

I felt so betrayed by my parents. How could they send me to this place? It was so awful. I didn't want to be here, but they wouldn't listen! I was so angry. I resented them for doing this to me. I felt so powerless and alone. I felt trapped in a place I hated. I never forgave them. I had lost yet another struggle.

On the other hand, I felt terrified of being abandoned by them. I was sure that being separated from my parents spelled doom. It was a Catch-22 situation. I wasn't safe with them, they still sent me to school, but I knew that I couldn't survive without them. I was dependent on them. I couldn't depend on myself for my survival. I had to rely on my parents for it, so I surrendered.

Soon after beginning grade one, my family moved to Little Britain, Ontario. I had already taken the same educational material in Nova Scotia's Kindergarten so I was advanced to grade two. (Ontario's school system includes grade 13. Kindergarten in Nova Scotia was equivalent to grade one in Ontario.) From then on, I was younger than my peers. I struggled in school. I couldn't concentrate and didn't want to.

But, at the same time, this was a new school — and a new chance. I had the opportunity to make new friends. My new teacher didn't know how shameful I was. I had a chance to belong, be liked and be happy. Soon afterwards, I got a small part in a school play. Although I didn't even have one line, I was happy to be part of it. Unfortunately, the play was a disastrous experience for me. I went out on stage before I was supposed to. Then when it was my turn, I was out on stage, beet red, terrified and very grateful that I didn't have to speak. After what seemed like two hours, but was only five minutes, I practically ran off stage. I was so relieved it was over. I felt so embarrassed. I felt way out of my element. I felt like the whole audience — it seemed like the world — had witnessed how incompetent I was. I resolved never to take up acting.

Living in Little Britain was fun. We lived in a beautiful big house with a huge yard where we could play tag and hide-and-seek. A couple in their eighties, Mr. and Mrs. Macleod, lived across the street. They would sit on their second floor balcony and watch the neighbourhood activities. They gave us candies every time we visited. I really liked them. I used to show off by riding my bike down the street in front of their house. Mrs. Macleod would tell me how good I was at riding my bike. One day my dad told us that we could no longer go over to visit because Mrs. Macleod had gone away. She had gone to heaven where she would be safe. I was very confused, and sad. I couldn't understand why she wasn't on her balcony anymore. I really missed her. I didn't like feeling that way and I didn't know how to handle it.

Our family moved soon after. By moving, I learned that if I move away from pain, I won't have to feel it. (Later, I often moved away from pain, a "geographical cure." Unfortunately, my pain moved right along with me.) Then we moved to Schreiber, Ontario for a year. During that year I had a serious bicycle accident that left me in bandages. I received an enormous amount of attention because of that accident. I loved it! I saw how much my parents really loved me. My parents dropped everything to take care of me. Even my much-loved piano teacher came to see me and brought me a board game as a gift. We played the game. I don't remember anything about the game other than my piano teacher chose a yellow player. Yellow has been my favourite colour ever since. I felt so loved by her, and by everyone.

Getting so much attention from so many people, I absorbed the message that, even though I'm not lovable, people will love me if I'm sick or hurt. All that attention made me feel good and erased my feelings of shame. After that, I did whatever I could to get attention. I even used to wish that I would become ill or injured (not too badly course!), so I could experience that attention again. I had learned how I could get attention and I had confused attention for love.

A year later, our family moved to Terrace Bay, only eight miles away. I was seven years old. I remember feeling very unhappy and insecure. I never knew when our family would move again. I missed my friends from Mahone Bay, Little Britain and Schreiber. During this period, my brother and I had many fist fights (which was not a smart idea since he was much taller and stronger than I).

One day I was in school and our class was given a reading exercise. Once the exercise was completed, students could listen to a story. All I wanted to do was listen to the story — I only wanted to feel good. I rushed through the exercise, barely completing it. Not surprisingly, I received a low mark. I hadn't even tried to do well. I didn't care about getting good grades. I only cared about feeling good. I felt awful, and very scared.

One night my parents had a party. They sent my brothers, sisters and me to bed at our regular bedtimes. I really didn't want to go, so I cried in bed. My mom came into my room and gave me a cookie. (I had fully expected to get a spanking or at least told to stop crying.) It was a chocolate-covered marshmallow cookie filled with coconut and strawberry jam. I could feel the love that came with that cookie. I knew that she didn't want me to feel sad. I ate the cookie. I had never enjoyed a cookie more. Later, I would often binge on that kind of cookie.

Soon after that day in class, my parents went on a trip to Toronto for what was to be one week. My father returned home without my mother.

A few days later, my dad took our family to a friend's house and there she was — my mom! I was extremely confused. I got an awful feeling in the pit of my stomach. I knew that something bad was about to happen. I was right. Our family returned home that night without my mom. She never lived with us again.

A woman who was a close and trusted friend of the family returned home with us that evening and stayed to live with us. When we got home that evening, the family, including our newest member, sat in the living room looking at travel brochures. We were going to be a happy family, a family who would travel and do all kinds of exciting things.

When my mom didn't come home, my worst fears materialized. I truly had been abandoned. All my basic messages were been confirmed. It sure felt as if I abandonment meant death; that I could never trust someone to be there for me and that I was definitely not worthy of being loved. I knew that I was truly a bad person — a good person would never have been abandoned, twice. Now, more than ever, I hated being this terrible, shameful person.

I didn't cry. I was in shock. I couldn't believe that all of my efforts to prevent my abandonment had failed. I had been abandoned, yet again. How this could have happened? I had done everything in my power to stop it.

I coped by focusing only on what I had to gain. I couldn't look back. I couldn't acknowledge that my mother was never coming back to me. Instead, I pretended it didn't matter. Then, I took action. My Head knew it was time for drastic decisions. So, then and there I resolved never to allow myself to really feel or grieve a loss, to quickly replace people and things as soon as they were gone, to never to trust that when people went away on a trip, they would return, never to count on someone to always be around, never to get too comfortable with life as it was because things would always change for the worse, and never to love someone completely. Most of all, I would never ever allow myself to be put in this position again!

Those decisions changed the course of my life dramatically. In effect, I decided to stop feeling. I split away from my Heart. I gave up myself, my feelings, my Heart. This way, I would never have to feel the loss of my mother. My Head took over completely. From this point, I lived safely in my Head, according to my thoughts, far away from my Heart.

I looked for a way to be safe. I figured that although my mother had left me, my father hadn't. Maybe I could be safe with him. I felt a different kind of safeness with my dad than I had felt with my mom, but it was safeness just the same. My dad became my protector, the person I depended upon for my survival. I decided that I had to do whatever it took to never be abandoned by my dad. He was my only hope for survival.

However, this time, I had to do it better. I had already failed to keep my mother — she had left me. My dad was still here, so I still had a chance.

I did my best to hide my "unlovable" self, my shame. Now more that ever, it seemed crucial to be perfect. I began to spend more time with boys and much less with girls. Soon after my mom left, I had my first boyfriend. I was eight years old and I was in love. I had never experienced such powerful emotions. It was so exciting. It was as though something wonderful was happening inside me. I felt so good that I didn't feel anything for my mom. I didn't even think about her. I thought that a boyfriend will make my pain go away. I wanted to be with my boyfriend, always.

I became aware of my appearance once I had a boyfriend. I remember walking down the street from my boyfriend's house, with baggy pants, feeling ugly. I never wore those pants again. One day, I was sitting beside my best friend and I noticed that my legs were much larger than hers. I felt absolutely gross. I was afraid that there was something wrong with my legs, they were so big. I was afraid that my boyfriend would be "grossed out" by my legs, and that he would reject and abandon me. From that point on, I was very aware of the size of my legs and would often compare them to others'. I felt relieved every time I saw someone with bigger legs than mine.

I was 10 years old and in grade six when our family moved to South Porcupine, Ontario. There was little talk about my parent's divorce. I welcomed that move because I could move away from pain, again. I could leave the house that reminded me of my mom, sitting beside me while I practised the piano, and sitting at our dining room table during meal-times. I no longer had to be in the rooms that made me think of her, the rooms where I missed her so much.

Although I wanted to leave those painful memories behind, I didn't want to leave two very special people: my best friend and my third boyfriend. My best friend and I did so many things together for most of the three years I lived in Terrace Bay. One month before we moved, my best friend and I had an argument that resulted in our not speaking to each other. We didn't resolve it before I moved. I believe I purposefully precipitated that disagreement so I wouldn't have to say goodbye and then miss her. I watched my boyfriend as he stood at the street corner while our family drove away in our stationwagon. I felt incredible pain. I wanted to jump right out of the car and stay with him. I felt so powerless, angry and sad. I didn't want to leave him, but I was powerless to stop what was happening. I just wanted to die.

I was 10 years old and had no idea what was happening to me. I knew that I couldn't deal with these feelings so I swallowed them. For the next 15 years, I felt the same pain every time I moved, or someone else moved away from me.

When we arrived at our new house in South Porcupine, there were boxes everywhere. Immediately, I got busy, unpacking boxes and arranging furniture. I wanted to feel comfortable, and fast. I couldn't stop moving or my feelings might catch up to me. I couldn't let myself miss my boyfriend. I couldn't let myself miss my mom. I had to keep moving.

Life in South Porcupine was filled with a lot of joy as well as pain. While living there, the family friend, my father's partner, moved out after having lived with us for five years, and once again, I didn't cry. I did miss her, but wouldn't allow myself to feel it. Now that my dad no longer had a partner, he had more free time and I saw more of him. I loved watching him cook, clean and take care of us. I was so happy when he would take us swimming, on a picnic, to the movies or out for dinner. With my dad caring for us, I felt so safe, so protected and so loved.

While living in South Porcupine, my dad sent my brothers, sister and me to camp for a few summers. (I hope all kids get to experience going to a summer camp. I'll always cherish my very special memories of it.) One day, I remember being in my cabin, lying down on my bed, and looking at my legs as I held them straight up. Again, I noticed that they were larger than the other girls. I worried that something was wrong with me. Why were my legs so big? I felt awful and different. I continued to look at other girls' legs to see if theirs were larger than mine. I asked my camp counselor if something was wrong with the size of my legs and she told me that they were beautiful. I felt a little better.

I had a boyfriend at camp. I asked him if he thought I was fat. He told me that I wasn't fat, but that I was bigger than most girls he knew. While we posed for a picture, I remember being very conscious of how large I looked. Camp ended and leaving those friends behind was extremely painful. I did not write or keep in contact with them. I couldn't be in contact with anyone that might bring up painful feelings. I would have had to experience them and I would not let that happen.

One day after we had arrived home from camp, I heard my dad say that it was nice to hear that sound again. He was referring to the sound of kids being home. He had missed us. I loved hearing that I was missed. I felt special. I felt loved.

I had been constantly comparing my skills to those of my friends, brothers and sisters. In most ways, I felt inferior. While everyone else was learning, practising and acquiring skills, I was withdrawing into myself. I felt very behind. I felt as though I had lost my step and needed to catch up. Yet I didn't know how. I was scared to move. I was the straggler who didn't pay attention to what the group was doing. I was in my own world, terrified to leave it and participate in the real world.

At the beginning of this stage, I was afraid that I was stupid, incapable and clumsy, but now I knew it. I realized that I didn't have the wherewithal to function on my own. I felt so shameful. When I did, I felt that "yuck" feeling in the pit of my stomach. I envied people who knew what career they wanted. I was sure that I was not competent enough to even try.

During this stage, I didn't learn intellectual, social or physical skills from educational material. I was focused on surviving. Instead, I learned that I was shameful and incompetent. I knew that I was a failure, and the pain of that feeling hurt almost more than being abandoned. I had to protect my Heart from feeling that hurt. I didn't care about being educated. I cared about surviving, and not being abandoned.

I ended this stage by feeling incompetent and inferior to others in every way but in appearance. In this area, I believed I had a chance. I figured that if I couldn't be smart, I could be pretty and slim. Already, people had responded positively to my appearance, although, I wasn't sure why. I didn't think it was anything special, but some people seemed to. I began the next stage with a mission. I was going to be the most attractive and the most irresistible young woman — and the thinnest! I devoted all my effort to making that happen.

Twelve

I SEARCHED FOR
MY IDENTITY

STAGE FIVE: Identity versus Confusion
(Age 13-18)

I *was in the basement. Two mattresses lay on the floor before me. Standing with great poise and confidence, I lifted my arms out high and raised my right leg out in front. Toes pointed gently toward the floor, I stood there, a beautiful, angelic gymnast. Integrating ballet with gymnastics, I performed my well-rehearsed routine. I began with a cartwheel, then a front walkover, followed by two graceful twirls, expanding into a back walkover, a backward summersault, unfolding into a handstand, completing my perfect performance by landing in the splits. I shot my arms straight up in the air. This was my routine. I felt so proud. I hadn't made one mistake. I could just hear the roar of the crowd. They loved me, absolutely adored me! For days, I had been trying to get a certain guy to notice me. Now, he was in the crowd, awestruck by my talent. I felt so special. I felt on top of the world. Not only did he love me, but so did everyone in the audience. Suddenly, I mattered.*

I was 12. I had never experienced that kind of exhilaration before. It felt so good and I wanted more. After it was over, I felt sad and lost. I did my routine again and again. I spent a lot of time practising gymnastics. I was hooked — hooked on feeling special, admired and loved. I adored this fantasy. I mattered. Then I began to act out my fantasy in real life.

Erik Erikson describes "identity" as an integrated image of oneself as a unique person. I had an image of myself as slim, beautiful and desirable, a fantasy image. In reality, I knew that I was just the opposite. I tried to forget reality. I could succeed when I was performing.

I tried to identify, to define who I was. In doing so, I experienced an "identity crisis", *a period of disorientation and anxiety resulting from difficulties experienced in resolving personal conflicts, adjusting to social demands and pressures.*[1] I wanted to be a unique person, a somebody, like no one else.

---

[1]Reader's Digest Association, Inc., p 837.

I wanted to be the best. I wanted to be different. I wanted to impress people. I wanted to be loved.

Adolescence is the bridge between childhood and adulthood. For me, being on that bridge was a terrifying experience. I experienced so many new things, so many unknowns. I experienced a great surge in my hormones and in my emotions. I experienced greater social pressure, like belonging to the "in" crowd, attracting men, and most importantly, being slim. I experienced high school, friendships and romances. I was very involved in sports. I experimented with alcohol. I went on my first diet. From my experiences, I learned how to become someone who is acceptable. I responded to this search with what was to become a 10-year-long eating disorder.

I was 13, and living in South Porcupine, when I first walked through the huge front doors of high school. What an experience! I was terrified and thrilled all at once. I think my heart stopped at that moment. I didn't know my way around and I knew very few people. I felt overwhelmed. I was too scared to even speak! But, I badly wanted to be part of all of this excitement.

I was painfully shy and nervous. I felt so incredibly inferior to everyone around me, yet I was determined to fit in. I had heard that if a person was pretty and slim they would be popular. If not, they wouldn't be accepted as part of the "in" crowd. I was so relieved to be attractive. I was willing to do almost anything to fit in.

How people saw me really mattered to me. Soon after starting high school, I began to notice that guys watched me (my peers and I referred to the males in high school as "guys"). Guys would stand along the glass wall facing the cafeteria, watching the girls walk by. They would watch us socializing in the cafeteria. I wanted them to see me as pretty and desirable. I would get so flustered and nervous every time I was around the cafeteria area. I always made sure to stop at the washroom to comb my hair and check my make-up, before I walked by them.

Being slim meant being accepted as part of the "in" crowd. Girls who were overweight were ridiculed and laughed at, often depicted as weak-willed people, unable to control their eating. I watched as they were shamefully rejected by my peers. I thought I'd die if that ever happened to me. I wouldn't allow it. I would make sure that I stayed slim!

I had been in high school for two weeks when I began my first serious high school romance. My boyfriend and I partied every weekend. I experienced the numbing and thrilling effects of alcohol for the first time. I couldn't believe how good it made me feel. This was the first time I had ingested a substance into my body that made me feel differently. I felt strong, confident and lovable. I loved feeling that way.

During the year I dated my boyfriend, I spent the days thinking about him in class, wishing the time away, and playing sports every day after school. On the weekends, I played in sport tournaments, I spent time with my boyfriend and my friends and I went to parties. My life was set — sports, boyfriend, friends and parties.

After that year, my relationship with my boyfriend ended, and another began. I was alone for about two weeks. This guy was even more special. I really admired him. He was older, wiser and extremely talented. He could play the piano and the guitar and sing. I was mesmerized. He was different from anyone I had dated previously. I dated him for the remainder of the summer and then he went away. Oh no! I couldn't handle my feelings. I was so mad at myself for having allowed myself to care so much. I thought I knew better. So I got busy. I did whatever I could to avoid my pain.

I discovered my love for sports in grade three. That year, I earned a badge called the Award of Excellence, the highest award in the scholastic physical eduction program. I had to complete a series of exercises, at a specific rate, that determined my level of fitness. For the next four years, I received that high award. After that, I participated in every school sport I possibly could. I learned to play basketball in grade six and loved it. I tried out for the team in grade seven, and made it.

By grade eight, basketball and other sports were a huge part of my life. In grade nine, my first year of high school, I tried out for the girls' junior basketball team, the best team to be on and the hardest one to make. Most of the players on that team were in grades ten and eleven. And I made it. I finally felt included, part of something. I belonged somewhere. In high school, I was considered a good athlete and gained a great deal of attention for it. My peers, other students and teachers, treated me differently, as someone special. I felt special, just like I had when I was a fantasy gymnast. As an athlete, I had found a very important part of my identity.

Since I was good in sports, I felt good when I was with my coaches. When they told me how well I had played, I felt validated, and worthy. I tried to play my best, to please my coaches. I wanted them to be proud of me. When I didn't play well, I felt shameful. I felt like I had let them down. So the next time, I tried twice as hard, not for my own joy but the joy I felt when they validated me. I was very lucky to have coaches who always validated and never shamed. None of my coaches ever yelled at the team to motivate us as many other coaches did. I felt competent and capable when I was playing in sports, with my coaches.

The guys who stood by the cafeteria also attended girls' basketball and volleyball games. So now, I brushed my hair and checked my make-up before each game. I really began to worry about how I looked on the court. I especially worried about whether I looked fat. I was more worried about how I looked on the court than how I played. My focus had shifted from what I was doing to how I looked while I was doing it. Then I began to worry about how I looked when I did other activities.

I worried about how I looked when I was in class, walking to and from school, and after school while at sports practice. I worried about how I looked outside school at the recreation centre where my friends and I roller-skated. I worried about how I looked in the park where a group of my friends used to hang out. I worried about how I looked at weekend parties. I worried about how I looked to my neighbours and finally, how I looked to strangers. I spent most of my time worrying about how I looked. The question I asked my sister most often was: "How do I look?" My appearance had become my main concern in life.

I was determined to find out what guys looked for in a woman so I did some research. I needed to know so I could work on fulfilling all the requirements. My research involved watching models on television, in fashion shows, and in magazines, questioning my male friends and my brothers and listening to how guys talked about girls. Finally, I watched how men reacted to women. I discovered their picture of the perfect woman. I concluded that men wanted a woman with Raquel Welch measurements (36-24-36), who was sexy, slim and preferably blond. They also wanted a woman who was outgoing, confident, kind, intelligent and athletic.

After I learned what men wanted in a woman, I tried to become it. Yet, I was severely limited. I didn't have a 36 inch bust — far from it! However, my waist was about 23 inches, so I had the 24 inch waist beat. (That was as close as I got to Raquel Welch's measurements.) I didn't have any curves. I was stick-straight. I used to wonder if I were supposed to be a male and somehow the chromosomes got mixed up. My body was a lot like a man's, and to this day, men's clothing fits me better than women's. I can joke about it now, but it was a major panic for me then. I was quite slim, but could have been slimmer. Thankfully, I was blond. (What was the big deal about being blond?) I wasn't smart — another strike against me. I wasn't confident or outgoing — yikes. However, I was athletic and I was kind. Overall, I didn't do too badly. At least I was still in the race! What a race it became.

I began to notice differences between my friends and me. Our body shapes were different. One night, when my best friend and I were at a party, I was absolutely crushed when the guy I really liked showed interest in my friend, rather than me. I felt so hurt and left out. Horrified by her betrayal, my friendship with her changed. She became the competition. I no longer trusted her or any other girlfriend.

After that betrayed, I felt like I had to compete with all other women. I believed that I could never let my guard down. I always kept close watch on how my boyfriend responded to other women, especially my friends. I felt inferior to women who were smart, confident, sexy, slim and had 36-inch busts. I saw them as very real threats to my survival. Those women had what I didn't, and I was extremely jealous. I was terrified that my man would prefer them and reject me.

I saw them as powerful, able to ruin my relationship. I saw them as people to fear and compete against rather than to relate with and enjoy. I became obsessed with making myself more attractive than anyone else. I couldn't stand to feel the fear of being rejected and abandoned by a man because he preferred another woman. To prevent that from ever happening, I began to eat less. I began to spend more time with men. I had fewer close girlfriends now. Women were competition.

In grade 11, I was captain of the basketball team, I was on the student council as the sports representative, and I had a steady boyfriend. I didn't think that life could be more perfect. I felt happy. I felt at ease. I wanted things to stay that way forever. I began to eat less. I hoped that if I could stay slim, things could stay the same.

Yet, I could sense that something was wrong, but I dismissed it. Then our basketball team travelled out-of-town for a weekend tournament. Throughout the weekend, I ate. My coach was very surprised by the amount I consumed because it was so much more than any of the other team members. I knew that I was eating a lot, but I couldn't help it. I was hungry.

Two months later, my family moved to Ottawa and I began to eat, voraciously. I ate as much as I had during basketball tournaments, only now I was at home. I just couldn't stop eating. I remember being in a restaurant with my friends, a few nights before I moved. All I could do was eat and eat and eat. In the middle of January, our family travelled to Ottawa. I ate constantly throughout that trip. I was surprised that I was eating so much, and that I never felt full.

I was leaving another boyfriend behind, and I had no idea how I would survive being apart from him. En route from South Porcupine to Ottawa, we stayed overnight in North Bay. That evening I remember lying on the bed, crying. I felt so overwhelmed with pain. It was excruciating; I couldn't bear it and I barely cared whether I did. The next morning at breakfast, I ordered pancakes. After I finished my breakfast, I ate my sister's breakfast, and then worried about whether I would get hungry while I was in the car. I just couldn't get enough to eat.

I didn't like my new high school. I couldn't be the captain of the basketball team — they already had one. I didn't like the building; it wasn't nearly as nice as my last school. The students didn't place as much emphasis on looks. I didn't want to be there at all. I was angry that I had to leave my boyfriend, my girlfriends, my friends and my sports. I felt lost. I barely participated in sports, yet I continued to eat a lot. My body was growing unattractively larger and so was my feeling of shame. I knew that I was growing even more unlovable, but I couldn't seem to help myself. Food made me feel so safe.

It was then that my father noticed my weight gain.

Our family was at a sports complex for a Sunday afternoon swim. As I was walking along the side of the pool, my sister commented: "Dad has just noticed how much weight you've put on!"... I just wanted to die. He could have noticed anything but my weight. Nothing could have been worse. Unfortunately, I knew he was right. I had gained weight — 15 pounds. I felt horrible, ugly, gross and definitely unlovable. I felt so terrified that he would reject me. Right then, I knew I had to lose weight.

I had gone from 125 to 140 pounds. I knew that I had been eating large amounts of food but before this I hadn't linked eating food with gaining weight. Before this move, I never gained weight no matter how much I ate. I had always been active in sports. This weight gain took me by surprise. I had been caught unawares and I hated that.

I felt like my shame had been exposed in the worst possible way to my father. If someone told me that World War III had been declared, it would have been less traumatic. I was absolutely crushed. I couldn't let my dad reject me. I had to get rid of this ugliness, this weight, and I don't care how I did it.

Although I was distraught, I knew what I had to do. I had to skip lunch. I skipped my first meal one sunny April day. I had arrived home from school with my siblings at noon. They were in the kitchen making sandwiches. I stayed outside. I knew that if I went inside, my hunger would get the better of me and I would give in and eat. My brother came outside and asked me why I wasn't coming inside for lunch. I replied that I wasn't hungry. Of course, that wasn't true, I was starving. Even more so, since I knew that I couldn't eat. Our lunch period was only 45 minutes, but it seemed like hours. I couldn't wait to be back on the way to school.

That afternoon in class, I was scared that I'd get too hungry. When I felt my stomach growl, I told myself that this was what I had to do. After the twentieth growl, I stopped feeling it. I was able to ignore my feeling of hunger for the first time in my life. After school that day, I arrived home feeling fine. I wasn't the least bit hungry. Even at supper time, I wasn't hungry. I ate very little. For the next two months, I skipped lunches and ate small suppers. I was getting good at this dieting. It wasn't as bad as my friends had made it out to be. Some of my friends were on diets from books, making specifically measured portions for each of their meals. I didn't have to do any of that. I was losing weight by the day. I lost 25 pounds in those two months. I was estatic.

Now, I weighed 115 pounds. I couldn't believe how much more positively men responded to me. I received approval and attention from many people, not just men. I had met a man when I weighed 140 pounds and I saw him again soon after I had lost weight. He was very impressed by how good I looked at 115 pounds. He had barely noticed me at 140 pounds. Now I knew that if I was slim and beautiful, people would love me.

To my horror, starving felt like torture — I couldn't handle the food deprivation any longer. I found myself eating huge amounts of food like a crazed animal who had gone without for days. I was eating so much that I had a constant stomachache. Now I was desperate. I was binging and couldn't stop, even though I knew what the consequences were — weight gain and rejection. I needed help, and fast. I couldn't keep eating like this. I tried to stop binging by taking diet pills but they didn't help — nothing did.

Then one day, I learned how to purge my food. I took a deep breath and felt faint with relief. I had found the answer. It seemed so simple, so obvious. I could eat as much as I wanted without gaining weight by simply "throwing up" food I didn't want to keep down. I no longer had to worry about gaining weight. Purging was my life-saver. I ended grade 11 with excitement. I could move forward in life without the fear of gaining weight. Unfortunately, I had no idea that I was beginning 10 years of binging and purging. I didn't know that what I was doing was called *bulimia* and I had no idea it would get much worse. I was binging and purging at least once a day. Other days, four times was not enough.

I quit going to school once I graduated, relieved that I didn't have to any longer. I wondered how I had managed to stay in school for as long as I did. I had hated it the whole time, but at least I had a place to go to. After I quit, I felt lost. My way of life changed. There were no more sports every day after school. And I missed my friends.

I lacked a sense of direction as well as safety and security so I turned to my boyfriend for them. I felt safe and protected with him, just as I had with my dad, even though I had only been dating him for a few months. Now he was my only sense of security; I needed him. I needed to ensure that he would never leave me. I needed to be slim.

Soon after, I moved from my parents' home into a house with my twin sister. I was afraid that I wouldn't survive out in the world on my own. Yet, I couldn't wait to leave home. I didn't want to answer to anyone anymore. I wanted my freedom. I had felt so shameful when I lived at home. I decided to face the consequences of being out in the real world.

I felt very confused. I didn't know what I wanted to do with my life. I was spending a lot of time watching television, talking on the phone, or partying at a nightclub. I felt ashamed about not doing anything useful with my life. I had little motivation to do anything. I just wanted relief from feeling like such a terrible person.

I desperately wanted to get attention and "wow" men so I took a modelling course. I was a model, out in the world, at 17 years old. I learned how to apply make-up and style my hair, how to dress, how to stand — all that was necessary to look good. Apparently, I achieved the desired effect because men were very impressed by the fact that I was a model. I was dying for attention. I was so happy that I had taken that modelling course, an indisputably wise decision.

One girl in the modelling class was told that she was overweight by 20 pounds. I felt so bad for her because I knew how she must have felt. I had been approximately the same weight before I had starved, binged and purged. I was so grateful that I had lost my excess weight. The sad part was, she was not overweight. She just wasn't "underweight," and therefore unable to model at that agency. Although not all modelling agencies require their models to be extremely thin, many do.

I chose activities that kept me in the limelight. As a model, I did fashion shows and photo shoots and had my picture in newspapers and magazines. I wasn't modelling because I enjoyed the work, but because I enjoyed the attention. I loved it when someone told me that they saw my picture in this magazine or that paper. I was modelling for the effect it had on others. I felt so excited and happy when I elicited a positive reaction in others, primarily men. I loved to generate awe. I was living my fairytale of being a fantasy gymnast.

Being slim was all I thought about. I put all my energy into my appearance. My body had become my identity and my worth. I weighed 115 pounds now and I felt worthy. I felt special. I looked good. At least I was doing something right. My absolute worst fear was that I would gain weight. I focused my energy toward enhancing my appearance and becoming slim. I read many books and magazines on dieting and food. I learned about what was fattening and nutritious, what caused pimples, and most important, what foods had the lowest number of calories.

The way my clothes fit shaped the way I felt about myself. A piece of material could make me feel horrible or incredibly happy! I felt on top of the world when my clothes were loose. Every time I lost weight, I felt so happy. Each time I lost weight was another chance to be loved. In contrast, when my clothes were too tight, I felt miserable. When I felt fat, I often punished myself by starving or binging. Shopping was another great way to get depressed. The mirrors in those change rooms were magnifying mirrors. They showed everything in gigantic proportions. When I felt fat, I felt like a failure. I felt only as good as I was slim.

When men were attracted to me, good feelings erased the shameful ones. Attracting men became my mission in life. I wanted to look better than other woman. I wanted to be the best. If I were the best, men would want to be with me and no one else. I couldn't run the risk of losing them. I had to be perfect so that they would never abandon me.

I identified myself with my body size. I saw no separation between me and my body size. (Just like I saw no separation between me and my shame and guilt.) I ended this stage in confusion. I was very confused about who I was. I concluded that I was a pretty, slim girl who modelled. I thought I was my exterior, my looks only. I didn't even know myself. What I thought I knew, I didn't like. I began to insulate myself from these painful and confusing feelings. I isolated myself from people. I withdrew from life and ate.

Thirteen

I
ISOLATED
MYSELF

STAGE SIX: Intimacy versus Isolation
(Age 18-25)

There, on the front page of the newspaper, was a picture of a boy, eyes wide, looking pleadingly through the bars of a prison cell. He had been quarantined because he was a schizophrenic. I stared at the picture in horror. I saw the tear on his cheek and my heart sank. Something shook inside me. I wanted to reach out to him, to somehow comfort him. I couldn't stand to see his pain. He was living my worst fear. Society had put him, a beautiful human being, away. I felt so powerless to do anything for him, and for me. I, too, felt like I didn't belong.

I would listen to the traffic, watch people walk by, and watch the day turn to night. Everything was moving, passing me by. I felt distant from the hustle and bustle of life. I knew I was wrong even to hope to be a part of it. So, I ate, again. I needed relief from this pain.

Erikson describes the task of stage six as developing *an ability to form close and lasting relationships; to make career commitments.* "Intimacy" is *marked by close acquaintance, association, or familiarity; pertaining to one's deepest nature.*[1] To "isolate" is to *separate from a group or whole and set apart.*[2]

I did not trust. I had not become autonomous. I was full of self-doubt. I saw myself as shameful, incompetent and inferior to others. I was confused about who I was. I was not about to become intimate with myself. I remained isolated.

In Chapter 5, "My Escape," I describe the ways in which I avoided and denied reality. It was during this stage that I lived this escape. Between the ages of 18 and 23, I tried to function in society. I had a job, friends and a steady boyfriend. Between 23 and 25, I withdrew. I no longer cared about my job, I stopped socializing with friends, and my relationship with my boyfriend ended. I lived in my own world of fantasy and food.

---

[1]Reader's Digest Association, Inc., p 879.
[2]Reader's Digest Association, Inc., p 890.

Leaving Food Behind

At 18, I was working as a retail sales associate in a successful specialty store chain. I loved my job. I could express my creativity through merchandising (displaying and positioning) clothes. I was beginning to feel good about myself. I was good at something. It had been a long time coming. I was promoted to assistant store manager and gained even more confidence. Then I moved to a department store and worked as a department manager. I could be even more creative. I was thrilled. I believed I was headed down the career path of retail management.

As long as I was performing well at my job, I felt good. But behind it all was the insidious fear that I would be found to be a less than satisfactory employee and let go. I was always scared of that. Although I tried hard not to be, I was besieged by the message: "I doubt you can do it."

I impressed many of my managers with my merchandising skills. I felt so good, so validated by them, just as I had with my coaches. I wanted their praise badly. Yet, I never felt truly at ease. I always felt as though I was just short of making it, just shy of perfection. I never let my guard down.

I disliked the way some managers treated me and my peers. I witnessed and experienced unfair and unjust treatment from one boss. Because I perceived this boss as superior to me and because I felt so shameful, I silently accepted this treatment, sure that I deserved it. When I became a boss, I made sure I treated my employees as equals.

I socialized with people who were attractive, and who appreciated the importance of good looks. I observed how they dressed, the cars they drove, and how they related to each other. I observed how the world responded to them. I learned what was acceptable, and what was not. I learned that sports cars and brand-name labels were acceptable and "Chevettes" and unknown labels were not.

I spent time at places where the emphasis was on appearance. I wanted my appearance (my identity) to be appreciated. I spent time at fitness clubs, disco bars, beaches, and any place I could experience the exhilaration of being appreciated for my appearance. I modelled and did fashion shows and photo shoots. I dated attractive men.

I was really uncomfortable when a person was more interested in me than in my appearance. I didn't know how to relate to them and didn't spend much time with them. I knew how shameful I was underneath my exterior. When they found out, they would inevitably leave me. I would leave them before they discovered that.

I loved to go running, teach aerobics and play tennis. I would often do all three in one day. I exercised to the point of exhaustion to have the perfect body. As well, I exercised out and away from my pain. Unfortunately, once I finished exercising, the pain returned.

I had been with my boyfriend since I was 15. He was strong, confident, smart, driven, organized, athletic and gorgeous. He was everything I wanted in a man. He was who I wanted to be. I depended on him completely for my safety and security. He was my lifeline. I was now 18 and he was about to take his first business trip. I thought that I was going to die. I hated trips. My parents had taken a trip, and it had ended disastrously — my mother left us, never to live with us again. Now my boyfriend, my lifeline, was going to leave me behind. I panicked. I went crazy.

After he left, my heart ached. I didn't know how to go on. As far as I was concerned, he had already left me behind. He was scheduled to be gone three weeks but came back after one. His early return didn't make a difference. To me, our relationship had changed forever. In my mind and in my heart, he had gone away for good. My message said that when people go away, then never come back. I could never again allow myself to love or care for him or anyone this much again. As though flicking a light switch, I turned off my feelings for him. Although we remained together for another five years, I tried to control my feelings for him. I grew more isolated.

I was obsessed with my relationships. They were my home away from home. They were my safety-line from danger. Whenever I realized that a relationship was unstable, I panicked. I tried to become thinner. I needed to ensure that my boyfriend would not leave me. Preventing weight gain was preventing abandonment. I felt that controlling my weight was controlling the outcome. I had to be in control so I dieted. It was a matter of survival.

Although the world of romance involved feeling safe, secure and loved, I knew that relationships didn't last. As exciting and exhilarating as they were, the pain they brought outweighed their benefit. I felt more pain than exhilaration. When they ended, I felt devastated. I felt as sad at the end of a relationship as I did at the end of a binge. I couldn't stand more pain.

As much as I hoped it wasn't true, I knew that I couldn't stop a man from leaving me. I couldn't control a man, but I could control food. My relationship with food became my primary focus — men were second. Food became the centre of my existence. Instead of waking up in the morning thinking about a man, my first thought was about food. Food never failed me, as all else had.

A new struggle began. Food was my dearest, most loving friend and, at the same time, a horribly cruel enemy. I felt so torn. I needed food. I depended on it to relieve my pain yet I had to deprive myself of it so as not to gain weight. Food helped me and hurt me. I felt betrayed by food, like I had by people, but I needed food. I chose to keep eating. What was happening to me?

I just couldn't see it. Eight years had passed — I was now 23. For five of those years, I had binged, purged, starved, and overeaten every day.

Yet, I denied I had a problem with food. I knew that I had not been eating normally, but there was no way I was going to stop. I couldn't. I justified my behaviour to myself. I rationalized that I needed food, just for today, and that tomorrow I'd stop binging.

I stopped purging when it became too physically painful. But, I continued to binge and quickly gained weight. My worst fear was coming to pass. So, for several months, I starved myself during the week and binged on the weekends. After a while, I forgot how much I hated purging and began again.

As soon as I was alone, usually right after work, I would sit in front of the television and eat. I would have already planned my meals. I would eat and eat and eat, until I was so full that I could barely get to the washroom. Beginning to purge was the hardest part, my stomach would be so distended. Yet I would have kept eating if I could have. I always felt so sad when a binge had to end. My fill of love was over and I could no longer make the pain go away. The pain would surface like a rocket — even sharper and stronger than before my binge. Then I'd purge, all that love, all that shame, all that wonderful and horrible food.

I didn't stop purging until it was all gone. Then I felt numb, completely numb. I had done it again. I couldn't believe it. I hadn't ever wanted to do that to myself again, but I had. It was as though someone else had done it to me, it was like a dream. It didn't feel like I chose to do this to myself. I had no control. I felt so sad and so alone. How could I go on living if I couldn't even control my own behaviour? I felt like I was really sick, a disgustingly horribly weak person. I was keeping a secret. Nobody knew about what I did in my apartment, behind closed doors, almost every night.

My struggle continued. I was searching, running, yearning for something. I didn't know what. I just felt empty. I was living a normal life by day and binging/purging by night. I felt such shame. I would go to work in the morning and return home at night, closing the door on the outside world. I couldn't stand to even walk to the store. I knew people would see right through me, right into my shame. I felt patronized, condemned, criticized, judged and disapproved of all the time now. When a teacher told me my work was unsatisfactory, when a boss told me that I was weak in a certain area, when a banker told me my credit card application had been refused, I felt incredible shame. I stopped trying to belong to society. I knew that I didn't.

On few occasions, I did get out. One day, I went to play tennis. Out on the court, I felt a wave of extreme shame wash over me. I felt totally uncoordinated and incapable of playing. I could just imagine what the people watching must have thought. I knew they would be disgusted. I felt so gross. I couldn't stand it. I just wanted to crawl under a table and disappear. At this point in my life, I felt that way often when I was out in public. I just wanted to die.

In actuality, I was living my greatest fear, that of being abandoned and alone. I was alone at birth and I was alone now. But, this time, I had chosen to be alone. I had decided that being isolated was safer that risking being hurt. I couldn't take any more hurt.

I was living an isolated life, estranged from others and myself. I had long since abandoned my own feelings. Now, I had closed the door on people who tried to be my friends. I wouldn't let them into my heart. I felt separate from everyone and everything. I felt left behind and forgotten. I felt very sad. I ate. I ate every time I felt lonely and I always felt lonely.

I believed that the world was a bad, hurtful and terrifying place. I wanted to stay hidden, safe within the confines of my apartment. I didn't want to live anymore. Though my pain and inner turmoil were unbearable, I was too terrified to feel it. I was certain I would die if I did. However, by now, I had little energy left to resist feeling. My pain was travelling quickly to the surface, like bubbles in boiling water. To keep them down, I ate as much as I could. I wouldn't let anyone get close to me, yet I desperately wanted help. I was completely isolated. For the first time, I knew that if I didn't do something, I would die.

I began my first step to leaving food behind. I began to feel. My recovery began.

Fourteen

THE
BEGINNING
OF MY
RECOVERY

Age 25

"*You're too sensitive. You overreact to everything. Don't say that, you'll hurt her feelings. Don't cry. Don't laugh. Keep your voice down!*" I couldn't escape the voices in my head. I had been walking along the river when I realized I was moving at a near sprint. My fists were clenched and my jaw was aching from gritting my teeth. I thought to myself, no wonder I woke up every morning with sore jaw muscles. I'd have no teeth left if I kept grinding them. I was so tense. I tried to relax but couldn't. I barely knew which way was up. I didn't know to feel. All my feelings were wrong. Why was I so sensitive, so sad all the time? I looked up to the sky for answers. It was dusk. The summer night was beautiful and warm.

I stopped walking, and stepping onto a large rock near the shoreline, I began to sob. I couldn't contain my feelings any longer. Losing control like this seemed wrong, but I couldn't help it. My feelings were exploding outward. I didn't care who might see me. I just stood there, weeping, feeling more powerless than ever before. I looked out over the river, watching it flow, as tears streamed down my cheeks. It felt good to cry, so good, for the first time.

I was overwhelmed by life. I had lost the struggle to keep my feelings down and inside me. I had no more fight left, no more energy to race home at night to binge and purge. That excitement had left long ago. My feelings gushed to the surface by the river. My recovery had begun.

That night, I felt emotions, strange emotions, *my* emotions. Surprisingly, I wasn't scared of them while I was feeling them. They seemed alien, yet familiar. While I was crying, I felt their warmth through my sadness. I felt close to something — to me — as I stood alone by the shoreline. Although a few people were nearby, they were far enough away so that I was all by myself, but I didn't feel alone. I was doing something that I had never allowed myself to do before, that I had stopped myself from doing, that I was terrified of doing — and it felt good! I was crying like never before.

Leaving Food Behind

I couldn't believe what was happening to me. I was filled with sadness, and, at the same time, tremendous love. For the first time, I realized I had been running from my feelings and emotions, fearing they were my enemies. I only discovered that they weren't because they had become too strong to suppress. Otherwise, I would have continued to run from them. I felt like I had been running from a loving soul who I thought was a bad guy. Only by running out of breath was the loving soul able to catch up to me, and only then, was I able to meet it and embrace it. I finally embraced me, my emotions, and my heart.

Experiencing my emotions that night by the river, I had such a powerful taste of what was inside me that I could no longer turn away from it. While my fear messages still told me that I couldn't feel and survive, my heart told me the opposite. I had been terrified of feeling for so long that I didn't know what to believe. My fear was overwhelmingly strong. My new understanding about my emotions was new and weak. I was afraid to believe that my emotions were my friends and a wonderful part of me. I faced a choice, an extremely important one. I could choose to believe my fear and continue to run from my emotions, or I could embrace my emotions and experience my pain.

I wished there were a third alternative. I weighed the pros and cons of both. I knew that if I continued to respond to my fear, I would carry on a miserable life of binging, purging and starving. My health had deteriorated badly. I had to drag myself out of bed every morning because I had either grossly overeaten the day before or was faint from starving myself. Either way, I had no energy. Then there was the depletion of emotional energy. Happy people had lots of energy. I was anything but happy. My sadness, anger, worry, shame and fear drained my energy like gravity drains water from a bath. I watched my energy swirl downward.

The alternative to feeling was grave. I felt as though I was between a rock and a hard place. Unfortunately, I needed to be in exactly that predicament, and experience that pressure, to be forced to choose. I had already exhausted all other alternatives. I faced reality and accepted my situation. I had an eating disorder. I was painfully unhappy. I knew I needed help. I accepted that I couldn't control my eating. I chose to feel my emotions. I can tell you today that I recovered from my eating disorder because I made this choice. By feeling, I recovered my ability to understand, validate, support and nurture myself. I learned to feel my heart. I recovered my true self. And *I left food behind*.

Food had become my best friend. I had isolated myself from everything and everyone. Food meant everything to me. Though I didn't like it that I binged, purged and/or starved to inevitably binge again, I wasn't ready to let go of food, not yet. Instead, I did the opposite. I ceased trying to stop myself from binging when I felt the need. I actually allowed myself to binge whenever I wanted. Also, I stopped punishing myself with shaming mental attacks after each binge. (I was so horribly cruel.) Although I didn't like it that I needed to binge and purge, I knew that one day, the need would disappear. I knew that food was not the real source of my pain.

My recovery continued. But, I thought to myself: What do I do now? Where do I go from here? Where do I begin? I didn't have a clue why I was binging and purging, overeating or starving. I was scared and confused. I paced my apartment while these questions went through head.

I left my apartment to go for a drive and I met a group of friends. Among them was a man whom I had met before, but didn't know well. I had no idea then how meeting him would change my life. He turned out to be a guide, a gift, that was available to me right when I needed it. I would learn where to go next — my new friend would teach me. My life changed dramatically, and for the better.

That night, I asked this man for help. He took part in a 12-step recovery program called Al-Anon (not associated with Overeaters Anonymous) and had "sponsored" many people. (A "sponsor" helps a member by guiding and teaching them the meaning of the 12 steps. A sponsor listens to and helps a person in need in times of trouble and pain.) He had never sponsored anyone with an eating disorder before.

I had never spoken about my eating disorder, or shared any other intimate facts about myself, with anyone. What I was about to experience was new to me and what he would learn about eating disorders was new to him. I could go to him at any time. I could count on him to be there for me. He did not judge me. I wouldn't be where I am today without his loving support. I needed a friend, and I had one. That evening, I was desperate for help, and there he was. (I don't believe in coincidences.)

A week later, I went to his home. We spent the first few hours talking about trivial things, then we got down to business. He asked me a question that took me aback: "How do you feel?" I was startled and bewildered. I couldn't respond. I thought to myself: "Is he talking to me? No problem, I can handle this question. Um. That's an easy one. Okay, I can tell him how I'm feeling. Um, um. Gosh, how am I feeling? Well, how should I feel?"

I couldn't believe that that one simple question could throw me into such a quandary. I felt like I was trying to speak a foreign language that I had once spoken and long ago forgotten. I had no idea how I truly felt. I couldn't remember the last time someone had asked me that question. I couldn't answer him.

I went home that evening, without having revealed my feelings to him. I wondered why I couldn't. How did I express my feelings? How will I ever be able to speak from my heart? I didn't know. I hadn't done it for so long. I stopped trying because just the thought of expressing my feelings turned my stomach. I felt such intense shame. My feelings actually repulsed me. I wanted to purge them. I thought: "I can't deal with them."

My next reaction was automatic — I wanted to run as far away from this situation as possible. I wanted nothing to do with any of it. I stopped myself right there before going any further, as though I had grabbed the scruff of my neck and pulled myself back. I had always run from my shame before. I had never tried to face it, until now. The feelings of shame that were directly associated with my feelings were so basic, so crippling and so familiar. But this time, I would give in to that shame. I was determined to feel, with or without shame.

Another obstacle to expressing my feelings was a desire to impress my friend. When I was with someone who mattered, I would allow myself to express only feelings that were acceptable or expected. I wanted him to like me, not see me for who I really was. I told myself that he really didn't want to know how I truly felt. He couldn't. Could he? I was so scared that he would leave me. But part of me knew that he really did want to know how I felt. I wanted to know too.

His question changed things for me. I couldn't deny my inability to describe my feelings. I could hardly describe something I wasn't in touch with. Stunned by this realization, I became acutely aware of how separate my feelings were from me. My "Head" and "Heart" were completely split; the wires had been disconnected long ago. I felt numbness and confusion. My first real moment of connection took place by the river.

So here I was, at the beginning of my recovery, ready and eager to begin feeling again, and I had no idea how. Was I crazy? Did I really want to open up this yucky, feeling thing? Could I really do it and survive? Was there still time to turn back? Then I saw my alternative staring me in the face, as I looked toward the bathroom and pictured myself purging. I knew I couldn't go back to that miserable life. I set out to reunite my "Head" with my "Heart."

The next step was to learn the definition of feeling. The definition of "feel" is *to experience (an emotion or condition); to be moved by or very sensitive to; to perceive or be aware of through physical sensation.*[1] I took a moment to absorb this. In other words, when I felt something, I was feeling a sensation, physically or emotionally. So when I felt happy, I felt the emotional sensation of love and the physical sensation of elation and lightness. Then I wondered what made me feel happy? So I looked up the definition of emotion. Emotion is (*e- out + movere, to move*) *a strong feeling; any of various complex*

---

[1] Simon & Schuster, Inc., p 497.

reactions with both mental and physical manifestations, as love, hate, fear, anger.[2] So, emotion was a response such as love, and to feel love, was to experience the sensation that love creates — elation and lightness. I feel my emotions. All right! I understood!

Two weeks after the first visit with my friend, I arrived at his doorstep once more, with tears streaming down my cheeks. I didn't know what was causing me to cry, but I was feeling! I stepped into his home, sat on the couch and began to describe, between gasping for breath and blowing my nose, how I felt. I didn't understand what was going on inside me. Words were few and far between. Mostly, I cried. Then, he held onto me like no one else had ever done. A while later, after I had stopped crying, he calmly asked me how I was feeling and I described a thought.

He told me he appreciated my thoughts but he was really interested in how I was feeling. I had such a difficult time answering him. I knew I was talking in circles, but it didn't matter. I kept trying to express my feelings. My friend kept listening and I went home that night feeling much better.

After that, I visited him much more frequently. Many of our conversations ended with tears and smudged mascara. Sometimes just trying to describe my feelings made me weep. I cried because I knew that he genuinely cared about me. I knew that he really wanted to know how I was feeling. I knew that he wanted to help. Sometimes, just his show of love and affection made me cry. I spent so many hours talking to him, the most valuable hours of my recovery. I am forever grateful to him.

I found it difficult to talk to anyone other than my friend. When I did, I felt intense shame wash over me. I wasn't comfortable discussing my recovery with anyone else. I was feeling very vulnerable, and I was vulnerable. I couldn't have handled it if someone had said anything hurtful about me. My emotional wounds were wide open and I needed time to heal. I knew that I was very lucky to be able to spend so much time on my recovery. I didn't have a family, children or a husband. I didn't even have a boyfriend. For the first year of my recovery, I spoke to few people other than my friend.

I filled a binder with blank lined paper and wrote almost every night. This binder, my journal, was precious to me. I expressed myself like never before. I had never allowed myself to think about, never mind write about, my feelings. I loved writing in my journal. Every night after I climbed into bed, I would pick up my binder and pen from under my mattress and begin to write. The content of what I wrote wasn't important. I wrote about anything I felt. I wrote about how I felt that day, about what a

---

[2]Simon & Schuster, Inc., p 445.

person said or did to me, about how scared I was — the fear went right down into the depths of my bones — and how sad and lonely I was. I wrote about how I felt about the special man in my life or how much I wanted to be with a particular person. I wrote about how bad and shameful I felt. I just wrote and wrote. I only wrote when I felt like writing. I never forced it.

I was surprised to see what I was writing. I was surprised at how someone's actions or words could bother me for an entire day, or even longer. A quick negative glance or a brief word was all it took to upset me. I was beginning to appreciate how sensitive I was. By writing, I really got to know myself. My words, through my pen, revealed deep feelings and emotions like hurt, hate, love and extreme sadness. Words were being written by me, yet I was as surprised by them as anyone.

My pen spoke in a way I could not. I felt safe when I was writing in my bed with my pillows and plush comforter. I felt like I could write about anything. I didn't have to worry about what anyone else thought. These words were for my eyes only. I expressed so much emotion in those pages. I let out anger, hurt, shame and fear. I described situations and my feelings about them. Although I didn't realize it at the time, writing in my journal was a way of releasing (purging) many of my painful emotions. Ironically, I resisted writing essays and other homework assignments during my school years, much to the dismay of my teachers. I was surprised that I enjoyed writing as much as I did. I was never that motivated before. Once I began, I was hooked, and I loved it.

I dated my journal each time I made an entry. About eight months later, I decided to reread some of it. But it was too soon. I was afraid that the fears and shame I had written about might be true. I decided not to continue reading. Those words were still too real, too possible. I decided to read my journal only when I felt completely ready, about a year later as it turned out. After that, I'd read a page every now and then. Many of my entries surprised me, providing great insight on how I had perceived life at that time. I could see that I was changing and growing. At times when I didn't think I was making much progress, I'd read what I had written just months earlier.

I wanted to recognize when I felt love, fear, anger, shame, guilt and sadness. To help me do this, I paid particular attention to their physical sensations. When I felt something, I asked myself: "Where am I feeling this emotion? Does it feel dull or sharp?" In this way, I learned how I felt physically when I was feeling shame, guilt, fear and pain. I tended to respond with the same physical sensation to fear, shame, guilt and pain — every time. I felt shame in the same place — in the centre of my torso, beneath my solar plexus, in the centre of my breastbone. Shame filled my stomach. My shame was always a dull sickening feeling of yuck. I wanted to throw it up (purge my shame).

Guilt was similar to shame, except that worry always followed. My whole body ached with worry. Fear was a sharp jolt in the pit of my stomach, between my solar plexus and my belly button. (Something like how I'd react if I were to face a grizzly bear!) When I felt sad, I felt a dull pain in my chest, near my heart. It was an ache that radiated through my body. I felt those physical sensations daily.

My body's ailments clearly revealed my emotions. I hadn't recognized those clues before. When I felt sick to my stomach, I felt shame. When I was sick of a person or a situation, I felt shame. When I was so angry I could just scream, I was angry! When my throat was constricted, I felt suffocated by my situation. When my muscles were tense, I was angry. When I was sick with worry, I was afraid. I held onto my emotions, unable to express them, so they manifested themselves in various parts of my body. I was sick — all the time.

I became aware of how I felt by the type of music I felt like listening to (rock, ballets or dance music); the type of book I felt like reading (Danielle Steele or Jack Higgins); the type of clothes I felt like wearing (casual or dressy); the colour of my clothes (red: fiery, assertive and confident, or green: natural and down-to-earth); and generally by my actions. When I felt the need to speed down the road in my car, chances were, I was angry.

I was drawn to the outdoors so I went for many walks. I felt a great desire to be close to nature, near trees and water. I loved to watch the sun sparkle through beautiful trees. I loved to see the sun's rays reflect on the ripples on the water, the little flowing waves formed by a soft, warm breeze. Nature was so alive. I felt its very powerful presence. I loved to listen to the birds sing. I had never appreciated birds before. I'd watch them fly. I'd see them land and I'd listen to them chirp to each other.

I loved to jog at my favourite spot beside a river. After my jog, I'd walk along, just watching the river flow. Everything was always so peaceful. The noise of the city was gone. I could hear my own thoughts and feel my emotions. Sometimes I cried. Other times I smiled. I never felt alone when I was in nature. When I was at home, I would look out of my bedroom window in the middle of the night and listen to the solitude of the night. I'd see the light radiating from the moon. Nature continued to sparkle.

For the first year of my recovery, I spent much time alone (or with my friend), learning to feel. I was gradually gaining the courage to let my emotions out. I wasn't sure what would come out but what would surface was very powerful. I felt anger, like never before.

Fifteen

ANGER

Age 26

Overcome with anger, I pushed the gas pedal to the floor. My Camaro Z28 shot out of the traffic like a bullet. The transport truck in front of me had been moving at a snail's pace, the pedestrian was taking his own sweet time crossing the road, the tourist beside me, checking his map while driving, had slowed to a stop at every corner. Everyone was driving me nuts! So my car and I bolted out of it. I had gotten away. But had I? I felt no relief. I was driving on the open highway, outside the city, yet I was still fuming. I grabbed my hair and tugged. I wanted to scream at the top of my lungs. I felt like I was going to explode at any moment.

I was furious. Until now I had been good at controlling my anger, but this time, it was too powerful. And that frightened me. I didn't want to hurt anyone with it. When I lost control in the past, I would smash my fist down on my car's dashboard, my kitchen counters, my walls or my bed. But, those instances paled alongside this. I tried, but I couldn't rationalize away this anger with my head. I couldn't reduce its force. There was no stopping it. "Just try to make it through the next few minutes without causing any destruction and you'll be okay," I pleaded with myself. I was still in my car, beginning to cool down ever so slightly.

I pulled off the highway into a park by a river. I got out of my car, steam escaping from my ears, and walked down the path to the shoreline. I looked out over the water. Everything was so peaceful. The birds were singing, unmoved by my anger. They seemed so happy. I shook my head as I was struck by the stark contrast between how I had been feeling moments earlier and the peacefulness and joy that surrounded me here. It was as though someone had just shone a spotlight on me and played back the last few moments. I saw clearly how overwhelmed with anger I had been. I had no idea that I had carried so much.

I hadn't realized that speeding down the road and cutting in front of other drivers was a sign of my anger. I did now! Before, I would have told myself: "If they hadn't been driving so slowly, so carelessly, I wouldn't have had to cut in front of them." Right? Wrong! But now, I realized that it was I who was driving too fast, too carelessly. I hadn't viewed a situation from this perspective before. I hadn't understood how I had contributed to, or affected a situation. I had always blamed the other guy.

Never before had I even contemplated facing my anger or my actions. I had taken one very huge step. I had no idea what to do with my anger or how to express it — without causing major destruction. This time, I was willing to learn. I didn't like having to feel my anger. I wished it would just go away. Yet, I still didn't run. I stood in that beautiful park feeling grounded among my whirlwinds of my emotion. I didn't know what was happening or what would happen to me, but I knew I was safe. Nature with its loving and calming presence had once again had given me incredible strength. I knew that I would never again turn away from my anger. I spent the next two hours sitting on a picnic table under a large maple tree, enjoying the birds and the stillness of the water.

Later that day, soon after arriving home, I looked up the definition of anger. "Anger" is *a feeling of extreme displeasure, hostility, indignation, or exasperation toward someone or something.*[1] That seemed right to me. I still didn't know what caused my anger, but that was okay for now. I went to bed that night, without injury.

The next morning I woke up with my nightgown drenched in perspiration. I opened my eyes wide in frightened confusion. I had just had a terrifying dream.

A man, whose face I never saw, but whom I knew and loved, was in an airplane. The plane was in mid-air over me. I was standing with another faceless man who was a dear friend. Suddenly the plane exploded. I stood in shock, not believing what I'd just witnessed. Flames and debris shot out, the explosion's deadly strength spewing shrapnel in all directions, including mine. The man beside me and I ran for our lives while an enormous fireball chased us. A split second before the debris and fire would have reached us, I woke up!

I had been dreaming about my anger. That's what the fireball symbolized. I feared that if released, my anger would cause horrific, devastating destruction. I feared that the energy release would be so powerful that it would kill me. I was terrified of my own anger. I had long forgotten that my anger was a natural, loving, protective part of me.

That morning, I was two months into my recovery. Here I was, trying to learn how to allow myself to feel, and I woke with that dream! Yes, I was feeling — feeling terrified. I was trying to accept my feelings, and now I was asking myself if I really wanted to accept this ferocious anger

---

[1]Reader's Digest Association, Inc., p 73.

that brewed inside me. My answer was yes. Despite the consequences, I was determined to acknowledge this fearful emotion. I knew that all of my emotions were a significant part of me, even the scary ones. I also knew that, at one time, my anger must have served me well. I made myself a cup of coffee. I needed one.

I felt more relaxed after my coffee, enough to ask myself what had provoked such vehement anger yesterday. I didn't know. I reread the dictionary definition. I felt extreme hostility toward something, but I didn't know what. Then I realized that I first felt angry after speaking to a "friend" on the phone. He had tried to make me feel guilty for not agreeing to have lunch with him. Hell yes, I was angry! I felt angry all over again just thinking about that phone conversation. I felt extreme hostility toward him for guilt-tripping me! He wasn't honouring my wishes.

I huffed and puffed, looking for a safe way to let this anger out. I had gotten so angry that I couldn't concentrate on work. I folded laundry, throwing each piece of clothing down onto its pile. A few hours later, feeling much calmer, I was back into my work when suddenly, I realized that my anger had been trying to protect me. My anger was meant to protect me from my friend's words. I formed my own definition of anger as the protective movement of energy-in-motion that responds to a perceived threat. My heart protects (feminine — protective), honours and establishes (masculine — assertive) my rights and safety. Anger provides its energy for protection from danger. Each time I felt angry, a threat was present, and I needed the protection of that energy.

One day, a few months later, I was shopping in a department store when I heard a mother yelling at her son. Within about five minutes, the mother said: "Don't give me any of that lip"; "Stop crying or you stay here"; "Don't you dare speak to me that way again!"; and "Don't use that tone of voice with me." The mother looked at me while shaking her head, as though to say: How do I ever put up with this? My look did not confirm her statement. Instead, I wanted to shout: There is a reason your child is crying! I wished the mother would give her child a hug, and tell him that it was okay to cry, and that mommy was there for him. Maybe that kind of loving response is easier said than done — I don't have children of my own. However, I understood the feeling of abandonment, shame and anger that child must have felt. (Even today, I cringe every time I hear parents relating to their children in that way. If parents knew how their words affected their kids, I wonder if they would still threaten them?) My heart ached for those innocent children. I identified with them.

I stood by the window that evening staring pensively into the darkness. I reflected back to my childhood, and the times when I had expressed, voiced or acted out my anger. I can recall being told: "Stop your yelling. Don't stomp your feet. You can go to your room if you keep acting this way. Stop your crying or we'll leave you here." It didn't take me long to realize why, as an adult, I had great difficulty expressing my anger. Those messages carried powerful and scary consequences for a kid, let alone an adult. I realized that my parents may have used those words as discipline tactics, but I heard them as real threats, with terrifying consequences. I believed them. I believed that they would have shut me in my room and left me there if I hadn't gotten rid of my anger and my angry behaviour.

When I expressed my anger, my bad behaviour was punished. When I expressed my happiness, my good behaviour was rewarded. I was no rocket scientist at the time. I didn't have to be. I knew what to do. I made a decision at that moment. I started internalizing my anger. I discarded one of my own emotions in exchange for safety — in my own home! I decided never to show my anger or my bad behaviour again. I had become a "good girl," behaving like a jewel.

I didn't allow myself to express my anger for years afterwards. I didn't realize the devastating effects that internalizing anger would have on me. Or maybe I did. At the time, the consequences of not doing so were far greater. Every time I felt the slightest hint of anger, I internalized it, right then and there. My head would intervene, inhibiting my expression of anger. I abandoned my own form of protection. My head had become my protector. (My head rarely got angry.) I did this for years, without realizing the process. I hadn't recalled making that choice until now. Now I understood.

I stood there, looking out the window. Though the night was dark, I could see myself, my life and my emotions so clearly and so brightly. I no longer wondered why I failed to stick up for myself with my friend yesterday. I knew now why I had said nothing to my "friend" to stop him from trying to make me feel guilty. I hadn't protected myself, fearing the consequences. His previous calls had followed the same pattern; he projected guilt onto me and I internalized my anger. Now I was feeling angry again, and it was okay.

I knew I had swallowed my anger because I was afraid of what would happen if I expressed it. But I didn't like what I started to feel next — anger and contempt toward my parents. I had been so vulnerable and dependent on them. I could picture myself as a young girl, so terrified of being deserted, that she had given up her anger, her only form of protection to survive, so as not to be left alone. As a young girl, I was weaker and more vulnerable than ever. Today, as an adult, I was feeling very protective of myself at that moment, and growing increasingly angry. I felt rage towards everyone who had ever hurt or threatened me.

So here I was, an adult, completely incapable of expressing anger when I felt it. I was completely unable to tell my "friend" that I wasn't interested in his friendship if it involved guilt. I couldn't communicate in that way — I had never learned how. At 25, I felt the same threat, the same fear of being abandoned by the person I was angry at, as I did as a child. In fact, every time I felt angry, I heard the message: "Don't express your anger, you'll be rejected and abandoned." My anger festered and grew inside me.

I tried to recall a time when I actually felt angry. Yes, there was one. I was 14. I had been yelling at everyone around me. At the time, I couldn't understand why I was feeling so angry. I was enraged. My father asked me what was going on with me. I was afraid he wouldn't like what he saw, so I decided not to curtail my angry around my dad, or anyone else who mattered to me. Instead, I swallowed it, and began to eat even more.

A few months passed. I received a call from a friend cancelling a trip we had been planning for months, at the last minute. I was really looking forward to this trip. I felt angry, disappointed and hurt, and I told her so. Although I thought I had communicated my hurt calmly, she didn't receive my words gracefully. In fact, she got mad at me for not understanding her reasons. Our phone call ended abruptly.

Soon afterward, I began to feel guilty. I couldn't believe it! I hadn't done anything wrong, I wasn't the one who cancelled, yet I was feeling guilty. I realized that expressing my anger had scared me. If I hurt my friend, then she might not want to be my friend any longer. I had been afraid that by verbalizing my anger, I might lose someone I needed and wanted close to me.

When I was young and unable to internalize it, I remember times my anger would come roaring out. I remember being told "to button up" or "to shut up" or "put a lid on it." I felt guilty for having been so weak as to be unable to "keep a lid on it." Those words confirmed that my anger was bad, shameful and dangerous. I knew that I needed to button it up, shut it up, or do something with it. I needed to do anything but release it, especially when my parents were around.

I felt like such a bad person for being so angry. "Good girls" don't get angry. When I was a child, I felt guilty for having destructive thoughts toward my parents. I didn't understand where my desire to hurt them came from. At the time, I had wanted to shed those horrible thoughts and feelings — immediately. But I couldn't. They were inside me. I had internalized them too. So, not only had I felt angry, I felt terribly guilty for being angry.

I wanted to accept my anger. Each time I internalized my anger, it was added to an internal reservoir of 25 years of accumulated anger! Only by now, it had become rage. I experienced this rage the day my Camaro Z28 and I bolted out of the city to that peaceful, beautiful park.

It was now six months since I had begun my recovery. I was feeling stronger and more able to accept my anger. I sipped on a cup of coffee, enjoying the warm breeze that was blowing through the balcony door. I looked into the large leafy tree that stood so tall in the backyard. I remembered times in my teens and early twenties, when I would get so angry I couldn't see straight. The slightest trigger could set me off. Those times gave me a taste of just how much anger I had internalized. With each explosion (thankfully there were few of them), I reinforced my vow to keep an even tighter seal on my anger. As well, those outbursts were short-lived. When my rage did manage to explode outward, I had control of it within seconds — my anger was internalized once again.

I had been in control — so I thought. I couldn't believe that I actually prided myself on being able to control my emotions. I used to feel so good about it! At this moment, I wished I had been much less able to control my emotions. I wished I had been too weak to internalize all this emotion. I would have had so much less to deal with. I turned away from the tree as though I was turning away from a wish that could never be. I had this emotion, this rage to deal with. I took a deep breath, attempting to draw in enough energy to face whatever would come next.

My appreciation of what resentment was and how it affected me, came next. I realized that I could feel worse than anger. I could feel resentment. I felt resentment toward a person who repeatedly hurt or disappointed me. I resented someone who repeatedly broke my trust. When I expressed my hurt, and they continued their hurtful behaviour, my resentment grew. Unfortunately, I held onto relationships that were hurtful and with people whom I resented, believing that I deserved such hurtful treatment. Yet I still resented people who hurt me. I felt like I was caught in a web of pain. I never got out of that web, even though the formula had been provided to me often.

I didn't get out of the web when I was young. The difference was I had no alternative. This time I thought I deserved to be mistreated. At least someone was around, I had rationalized. However, mistreatment was no longer acceptable. I was better than this, I thought. I knew that no one deserved to be treated badly, invalidated, laughed at, put down or yelled at. I was in my apartment, alone and happy to be alone. I had spent the last six months away from people I had spent much time with. By being away from them and other distractions, I felt more peaceful, less defensive. I didn't have to justify what I was doing, feeling or saying to anyone. I needed this time alone. Seven months had passed since recovery had begun. Every day I was growing one step closer to myself, my feelings and my emotions. I had grown away from most of my friends. I needed that separation.

I reflected on one particular relationship. It had begun blissfully and ended in hurt, anger and resentment. In its final stages, I had felt nothing but contempt and resentment for a man whom I had initially trusted. I realized that beginning to resent him heralded the end of that relationship. My feelings of resentment were toxic and destructive. I became very unkind to him, putting him down at every chance. I felt like I was at war. I felt no love for him, only disgust. I held onto resentment toward people who had abandoned me, emotionally, physically or mentally.

It was always so exciting to meet new people because these were people who hadn't yet let me down. I had no negative feelings toward them. I used to wonder why I would be so willing to do something special for someone I barely knew, and not for those closest to me. Now I knew why. I related to someone new with energy and excitement until they let me down or hurt me. When a person proved to be untrustworthy, I withdrew from them emotionally, feeling resentful. Then I would meet someone new, and the process would begin again.

I couldn't tell my "friend" that his guilt trips weren't appreciated. However, I could jump in my car and tear down the street, cutting in front of other drivers. I had displaced my anger toward my "friend" and projected it away from the source onto the other drivers on the road. It was safer to be angry at them; there were no consequences. One day when I was young, my parents told me that I couldn't have a doll I wanted. I got very angry at them. I couldn't express my anger to my parents, but when my sister received a doll, I called her names for two days. My sister was not the source of my anger, but I displaced my anger onto her. I had been displacing my anger for years.

For years, I had projected a great deal of anger onto many people, instead of directing it toward the real source. I had so much rage and resentment brewing inside me that needed an outlet. I broke things, hurt and manipulated people. I displaced my anger by calling people stupid, dumb, pathetic or deaf. In my adult years, I gossiped and judged people cruelly. I hurt many people by my words and actions. I had lashed out, intending to hurt, just like I was hurt.

I manipulated people by taking things from them without asking. I had relationships with certain people for my own gain. I gave to others what I thought they wanted so that I could in turn, receive from them what I wanted. I passively expressed my anger to close friends and family by not doing favours, by not confiding in them, by not helping them when they asked, by not contacting them. At work, I expressed my anger by doing less than a satisfactory job, forgetting important dates, and generally disappointing people.

When I was with a person at whom I felt angry, I would feel sick to my stomach. I would not care to talk to or to spend time with them. (Unfortunately, I felt angry toward the world and felt sick all the time!) When I was feeling anger toward my partner, I could not be intimate with him (physically or emotionally). I was feeling anger, not love.

I was angry for so many reasons. I was angry at others and at myself. I was angry because I wasn't allowed to express my anger. I was angry that my parents had threatened me so many years ago. I was angry that my parents had yelled at me instead of hugging me. I felt angry for feeling abandoned by my parents. When I was told to stop crying or I can go to my room, I felt abandoned, emotionally. When I cut my knee and was asked why didn't you look where you were going, I felt abandoned. When I felt angry and was told to button up or else, I felt abandoned. I was very angry that I had been abandoned and felt so alone. I felt utterly helpless. I could scream, shout or cry and it didn't help, nothing helped. Actually it made things worse. No one heard me. No one listened. No one cared. I felt terrified, angry and alone.

I had not run from my anger. I was so grateful; it would have been so easy. I understood that I had internalized it. I was beginning to realize that giving up ("addiction" — *to give up*) my own form of protection had a great consequence. I had become dependent on other people for protection. I wanted to cry and cry and cry.

Sixteen

GRIEVING

Age 26

t was the middle of the night and I was looking out the window. I was watching the cars go by, the glow of the street lights and the wind blowing against the trees. The moon was full, and so was I — full of sadness. I wondered what life was all about. I wondered why I felt so alone in this populated world, alone even in the middle of a crowd. I longed for love and companionship. I longed for a special someone to share my life with, someone to love completely. I wanted someone to walk the dog with, to come home to after a long day of work, to have enthralling discussions with, to share my challenges, joys and fears with. I wanted someone I could trust implicitly. I wanted someone beside me when I awoke after a bad dream. I took a deep breath and sighed. I knew no such person. It was just as well, I thought, no I minimized. I rationalized that I couldn't take any more hurt — relationships were too painful anyway. I continued to admire the moon on this peaceful night. Then, I felt something stir inside me. The feeling gained strength, and within seconds, I felt my emotions erupt. I began to cry. I wept and wept and wept. I had begun to grieve.

Here I was, seven months into my recovery, I thought, wiping tears from my cheeks. This was the third time I had cried like this. I reviewed what I had learned thus far. I understood what feelings and emotions were and I knew that I had rejected and abandoned mine. I realized that I had a great deal of anger inside me. By now, I had experienced my emotions by the river, with my friend, and now in my apartment. I knew by the depth of the sadness I had just felt, that I carried as much hurt as anger. As I stood in the middle of my apartment, I felt as though I was in the middle of a three-ring circus. I was desperately trying to make sense of what was happening to me.

I tried to figure out the meaning of this sadness. My crying outburst had been brought on by feeling the absence of a special someone in my life. I felt a very real and painful sense of loss — something was missing. Yet, that sense of loss seemed familiar. I had felt it every day of my life, if only for a fleeting second, before I pushed it away. That feeling was of missing someone, possibly more than one person, that I had been close to and cared for deeply. I didn't know the specifics, such as who it was, or when the separation had occurred. But, I was so happy to have this much understanding, however slight it was, of the meaning of my emotions, instead of just being overwhelmed by undistinguishable pain. The process of feeling had begun. I went to bed, exhausted.

I woke up the next morning feeling very afraid. I was afraid of letting go of this pain. My painful emotions were like old friends, not pleasant friends, but familiar ones. In an odd way they were comforting for having been inside me for so many years. I wanted to unleash them but feared what would happen if I did.

Little did I know that I was about to make a critical discovery, and learn something that had never before occurred to me. One evening, my special friend asked me whether I had ever grieved the painful changes that had occurred in my childhood. I looked at him as though he were crazy. Of course I didn't need to grieve — no one had died. He suggested that I dig up some information about grieving. The next day, reluctantly, I went to the library and found a book called *Live with Loss* by Kate Walsh Slagle.[1] As soon as I returned home, I began to read. I read each page, each line, each word with my eyes wide and mouth gaping. He was right. This was exactly what I needed. I really needed to grieve.

I had finished half the book before I realized that day had turned into night. I was enthralled by the book and its contents. I put it down and looked up the dictionary definition of "grieve," which is *to feel deep, acute sorrow or distress; mourn.*[2] The definition did not surprise me, it was how I had perceived grieving. However, I had also associated grieving with death. Only by reading Slagle's book did I realize that death need not occur for grieving to be necessary. I defined for myself the meaning of grieving as to feel, to allow the flow of emotions in response to change.

Changes, not deaths, had occurred during my life. Change was the difference between what was and what is. Many changes had affected me as deeply as if they were deaths. I needed to grieve the painful changes. When my mother left our home, she hadn't died, but I still needed to grieve her loss.

---

[1]Slagle, Kate Walsh, *Live with Loss*, (Englewood Cliffs, New Jersey: Prentice-Hall, Inc., 1982). *The description of information that was derived from Live with Loss is a reinterpretation by Sheila Mather. The description may not accurately reflected that of the text found in Live with Loss.*
[2]Simon & Schuster, Inc., p 593.

I recalled nights when I would lie in bed pretending that my mother was dead. It was only then I could cry. When I stopped pretending she had died and acknowledged that she was still alive, I was no longer able to cry. I wanted to feel her absence but I couldn't. There had been no finality, no death. I hadn't been able to feel my pain because I hadn't understood, why, if she were alive, she wasn't living with me. She hadn't died. I hadn't grieved.

One day I was playing hide-and-seek with my friends and my greatest concern was finding a place to hide to avoid being found. Three weeks later, everything had changed. My mother was gone. She had left us and was now living at someone else's house. Now, my greatest concern was how to go on living without my mom. At seven, my family, my roots, my grounding had completely disintegrated. The foundation that had existed was now gone. I was in shock. One minute I was playing hide-and-seek — a joyful and playful seven-year-old. The next minute I was living without my mother. If this was change, I hated it.

One evening, when I was about 14, my father told my brothers and sisters and I that my dog had been killed — she had been hit by a transport truck. I felt as though part of me had been ripped away. I loved my dog. I loved to come home from school to be greeted excitedly by her. I loved to take her for walks. I loved to watch her run and play in the field behind our home, investigating every tree, shrub, hole and stick. She was so curious. I didn't understand why she had been taken from me. It just wasn't fair. My dog was gone and I couldn't do anything about it. I so desperately wanted to change what had happened, but her absence was final. I felt hurt, sad, angry and helpless. One minute she had filled me with love and the next minute, she was gone. I had been out playing with my friends when she was killed. I had no idea what would await me when I got home that evening. If only I had stayed in that night, I thought, she wouldn't have gotten away and run across the highway. I could have saved her, but now it was too late. If only I had been a better daughter. If only I had known that my mom was going to leave, I could have stopped her. I was devastated. I hated change.

My perception of change was loss and pain. My world changed when my dog died. My world changed when my mom left. My world had changed when our family moved from South Porcupine to Ottawa. Change was loss. Change was painful.

One beautiful, sunny, spring day, I went for a walk by the shore of a river. The sun was shining warmly, the river was flowing and the branches of the trees were swaying with the wind. I could feel loving energy radiating from nature. I looked around me and wished with all my heart that time would stand still — that this day, this time, would never change. I wanted to stop the traffic. I wanted to stop everything. I wanted to hold onto the beautiful feelings. "Why does everything have to change?" I asked myself. Why had our family moved so often? I didn't want to move ever again. I wanted to prevent any more changes from happening. I couldn't take any more. I felt so sad and so frustrated realizing that change was inevitable. That meant pain was inevitable.

Elizabeth Kubler-Ross, known for her work on grief, wrote a popular book called *Death: The final stage of growth.*[3] which I found very helpful. I found *Live With Loss* and *Death: The final stage of growth* at the library. Since then, I have read many other books on grief. I'm so grateful to have learned about grieving. By learning about the stages of grief, I could finally make sense of my chaotic emotions. As well, I was much less afraid to feel them. I felt comforted by knowing that my emotions followed a natural cycle. Below, I briefly describe the stages of grief presented in these books in my own words. I recommend these books to anyone who is searching for answers about the natural human response to change — grieving.

I determined from Slagle that there are three general stages of grief:

1. Shock and denial;
2. Disorganization, which includes searching and denial; depression, defeat and despair, anger and guilt, acceptance and;
3. Reorganization/restructuring.
    Here are my brief descriptions of each stage:
1. Shock and denial: The numbing effect which neutralizes the effect of the loss that acts as a cushion, allowing time for the person to become aware of the loss;
2. Searching: The person searches for the person or thing lost, hoping to find it at any turn;
3. Pining: finding the reality of the loss, pining down the truth;
4. Depression:
    a) defeat and despair: an overwhelming sense of helplessness
    b) anger: something has been taken away, they left me alone
    c) guilt: how can I be angry at my loss?
5. Acceptance: living with the reality of the loss, letting go of the loss;
6. Restructuring: new behaviours are learned; growing from the loss; life is put back together.

---

[3]Kubler-Ross, Elizabeth, *Death: The final stage of growth.* (New York, New York: Simon & Schuster, Inc., 1986). *The description of the stages of death and growth is a reinterpretation by Sheila Mather and may not accurately reflect that of the text in* Death: The final stage of growth

While reading a book called *"Further Along The Road Less Traveled"* by M. Scott Peck, M.D., I saw Kubler-Ross's stages of death and growth listed as:

- denial
- anger
- bargaining
- depression
- acceptance[4]

I experienced these stages as:

1. Denial: failing to acknowledge reality;
2. Anger: feeling out of control;
3. Bargaining: trying to reason with or work out an explanation about why the loss occurred, enabling the person to regress back to anger or denial;
4. Depression: having not found a explanation about the loss, having faced the reality, experiencing a feeling of defeat and despair and helplessness; sadness and pain and;
5. Acceptance: the loss is gone and it's okay. I can begin to live again.

Although these books outline a similar, but slightly different order, I grieved in both ways. I had many opportunities to experience each order. Overall, I was grateful to know that in whatever order I experienced my emotions, I was feeling them according to what was right for me. As well, I knew that I was following a process of grief to acceptance, not to insanity.

Change includes opposites such as: gain and loss; joy and sorrow; sunshine and rain; pleasure and pain. Grieving is an emotional response to change that involves travelling (feeling) through different emotions (stages) to accept that change.

By not grieving, I had stopped the natural flow of my emotions and prevented my wounds from being cleansed. By not grieving when my mother left, I had swallowed that hurt and carried it. I was saturated with emotions from losses I had not grieved. The burden of carrying all these was extremely heavy. By not grieving when my dog died, I carried that pain too, and responded to it daily. Every time I saw a dog like mine, I felt the loss. I couldn't appreciate any other dog. Every dog "symbolized" (*something that represents something else*) pain and loss. Every mother symbolized pain and loss. I was unable to love or care for anyone or anything.

Up to and including that day, at age 26, I had experienced many changes and losses. Not only had dogs and mothers become symbols of pain, so had boyfriends, friends, houses, towns, cities, cars, colognes and songs. The boyfriend and friends I had left behind; the houses I had moved

---

[4]M. Scott Peck, M.D., *Further Along the Road Less Traveled*, (New York, New York: Simon & Schuster, 1993), p 63.

from; the towns and cities I had moved from; the places I had visited and left; the car that resembled the one I had stolen; the colognes worn my boyfriends; and the songs that had been playing during happy times — were all painful symbols.

My days had been filled with painful responses to those things and more. I'd wake up in the morning to birdsongs and think of how my boyfriend and I used to listen to the birds in the morning. On my way to work I'd see a car like the one that I had stolen from me and feel sad. At work I'd smell a certain cologne and remember my ex-boyfriend and feel sad. I might hear a song on the radio that reminded me of another time, a happier time and feel sad. By this point, I was not responding to reality, to things as they were. I was responding to symbols of ungrieved changes. Almost everything and everyone in my life symbolized pain. I went from one painful memory to another.

I was exhausted by constantly feeling the pain that certain symbols (messages) triggered. Feeling the old, familiar pain helped me avoid facing painful changes in the present. The old pain cushioned me from new pain. I didn't handle the old pain well — I certainly couldn't handle new pain. I had been stuck, unwilling to step out of my old pain and face it — until now.

Learning how to grieve was the easy part. Now it was time to do what I had learned. It was time to release my emotions. It was much easier for me to think than feel my way to recovery. I wished that I could just understand why I was the way I was, and then recover without having to suffer the pain of grieving. Yet, the pain was worth it — I had already missed too much of life because I was scared to feel.

There were so many changes that I needed to grieve. To recover, to look forward to the future, I knew I needed to grieve. I needed to accept my past. Acceptance is the last stage of grief. It was time for me to feel, to pass through the stages of grief. I had been stuck too long in my childhood emotions. I was about to grow up emotionally. I was ready to become an adult, a whole person.

Seventeen

MY WAREHOUSE
OF EMOTIONS

Age 26

I had finally finished the report. I had worked very hard on it and I desperately wanted my friend to read it and give me his feedback. I asked him twice. He promised to read it when he was finished what he was doing. I waited. He forgot. I was heartbroken. Twenty-four hours passed and he still hadn't read it. By this time, I felt so hurt and angry, I couldn't see straight. I had trusted him. I thought he cared. How could he have just forgotten? I knew why, I had gotten the message, as my hurt and shame came exploding to the surface. I wasn't worth his time, his care or his love. I knew that I had no right to even ask, but I still felt hurt.

Finally, very angrily, I asked him when he thought he might have time to read my report. Nonchalantly, he said: "Oh yeah, your report. I guess I forgot." I saw red! I couldn't believe that he had "just forgotten," much less treated it as a mere oversight! I reminded him that I knew that he knew how much it mattered to me that he read my report. He confirmed that he did. Then I asked him how he could "just forget." He couldn't give me an answer. So I gave him mine. I told him that I knew that he didn't really care about me, that he didn't truly love me, and that he didn't see me as enough of a priority to take ten minutes to read my report! He disagreed with my conclusions, but I knew that they were right! In fact, I had known all along.

I knew that I had been fooling myself by hoping that he really did care about me. Even so, having my shamefulness and unworthiness confirmed was excruciatingly painful. I left the room, slammed the door as hard as I could, and ran into my bedroom. I crouched down pressing my back against the side of my bed, my arms crossed over my stomach. My head went back, as I was racked with pain. I began to sob uncontrollably. I felt overwhelming shame. I knew that feeling well. I had felt it so often as a young girl, as a teenager and now as an adult. I cried and cried. I was feeling so much pain. It was the same pain I had felt years before when I just wanted someone to take the time to read my work, to watch me play basketball, to look at my drawings, to be interested in what I *was doing, to care about me when I was scared, and to say it was okay when I made a mistake. I so desperately wanted someone to truly care for me. I wanted to matter to someone. But no one cared about me.*

I cried for what seemed an eternity and then stopped suddenly. I just sat there on the floor beside my bed, stunned. In that 15 minutes, I had just lived through the shame that I had been carrying for a very long time. Now, I felt different somehow. I no longer felt unlovable. I immediately went to my friend and asked him if he really loved me. He said he did. I asked him if he cared about what I did. He said he did and reminded me of the many times he had demonstrated his love and his care. I couldn't argue with him. I knew he was right. Before this, I wouldn't have believed him. Yet, he was the one person (other than my sister) who had supported me throughout my recovery. He never shamed me. He never expected nor wanted me to be anyone but me. For the first time, I realized that he did love me — unconditionally. For the first time in 26 years, I felt like I deserved it.

That experience was the turning point for me. It happened nine months into my recovery. It was my friend's complete and unconditional love that forced me to see that others had not loved me in that way. I wanted to do anything but face the pain that I had not felt unconditionally loved before. (I know now that my parents had loved me. It was just that when I was young, I hadn't been able to receive that love in the way that I had wanted and needed it.) I had held both my friend's love and my past pain, at arms length. But my friend loved me too much — I couldn't doubt him any longer. I had to face my pain.

That evening, my friend's actions and seeming lack of concern had triggered my pain and feelings of shamefulness. By feeling that pain, I had finally let go of a heavy chunk of the pain I was carrying. For the first time, I came face-to-face with the message I hung onto from birth that I was shameful and unlovable. I faced it by feeling it, and by feeling it, the message disintegrated, just like that. I no longer felt unlovable. I was amazed. It was that simple, and that painful. I only wished that I had faced it sooner. I could have been living free of that pain for all those years.

Yet, in fairness to myself, I understood why I hadn't faced that message sooner. I don't believe that I would have been able to experience that pain fully by myself. It was much too scary to face alone. Now I had my friend's support and love. I had confidence in his love and support. I knew I was safe to face and feel my pain. I could go deeply into it and experience it until it was completely gone.

I had been mired in suppressed grief for a long, long time. I knew what defeat, despair and hopelessness felt like. I lived with them every day. I considered the turmoil I lived with inside me normal. Feeling fear each morning when I woke up was normal. Being wildly jealous when my boyfriend looked at another woman was normal. Spending most of my time thinking about how I would lose more weight was normal. Spending a weekend obsessing about a special man was normal. Struggling to make people like me was normal. Failing was normal. Not crying was normal. Responding to other people's needs instead of my own was normal. I could expect and anticipate pain and disappointment — that was normal. But feeling, now that was not normal!

Living without the message that I was shameful and unlovable was not normal. I felt lovable for the first time. I was thrilled. I felt happy and free. But it didn't last long. I began to doubt whether the message was really gone. Maybe it was just my imagination. Maybe I was just fooling myself. Maybe it was going to sneak up on me and catch me off guard. Then I thought about all the other messages I had yet to face, and felt overwhelmed. I wanted to run back to safety, to where I had been before I faced the message. At least then I knew what to expect from life. Now I felt out of control. I didn't know how to handle not feeling unlovable, if that was indeed true. I felt lost.

Within minutes of feeling happy and free, I had worked myself into a panic. I knew terror. I did not know happiness. I went to my friend and told him about my fear. He told me that I had just stepped from, as he put it, a "warm and fuzzy" (normal) place and stepped into "cold and unfamiliar" (unknown) territory. He also told me that my new approach was like a new muscle, it was not yet strong. With practice, he said, it would grow, and as it grew, my fear would dissipate. I understood and felt somewhat less fearful, but I was still sceptical. This was all so new.

Two months passed. By now, I was visiting my friend daily. At some point during each visit, I found myself crying helplessly in his arms, for anywhere from 10 minutes to half an hour. I began grieving many of my past experiences, one by one. On this particular night, I had a dream.

I was standing at the entrance of a storage room in the basement of a large building. The room was full of cardboard boxes. Many unopened boxes were stacked from the back to the front of the room. At the front of the room, empty boxes lay overturned and sideways. Others were piled on top of each other. Some empty boxes had fallen out through the doorway into the hall, preventing me from walking past. I tried to close the door, without success — the empty boxes were in the way.

Then I woke up. It was the middle of the night. I wrote down the dream and grasped its message immediately. I had unpacked (grieved) some boxes (my most recent experiences) that lay empty at the front of the room. I needed to open up and clear out the remaining boxes to walk down the hallway (move on in life). I understood what was required of me. After I thought about this dream and its meaning, I took a deep breath and vowed to continued to unpack (and to feel) each box, one by one. I wanted to settle into my new home — myself. I closed my eyes and went back to sleep, feeling very peaceful.

After that dream, I saw the pain inside me as being in boxes — boxes that I had carried for a long time. I could picture how, as a child, I had handled painful experiences. Not knowing how to express my emotions in an acceptable way, when I experienced a loss, I packed it away. The boxes I used were similar to boxes supplied by a moving company. The difference was, my boxes were for the storage of emotions, not household items. When I experienced a loss, I placed my painful emotions into a box, closed it and sealed it tight, using extra packing tape. I wanted no part of them.

I then labelled the box according to what the loss was, when it happened, and put it in a warehouse. This warehouse was a long narrow storage room with one door. The boxes were stacked in chronological order. The boxes closest to the door were my most recent experiences and those at the back were my earliest. Each experience had its very own box; my warehouse was full. By the time I had my dream, I had opened and emptied many of the most recently packed boxes, but many boxes still remained to be opened. I was scared, but I pressed on anyway.

What surprised me most was my initial reaction to a box when I opened it. Each time I looked into a box, I would respond to its contents as though I were the age at which I had packed it. I was 14 years old when my dog was killed. When I unpacked the box labelled "Keltie died, 1979, Sheila age 14," I was 25 years old. Yet, when I felt the emotions in that box, I felt as though I were 14. I felt the same intense pain and sadness, and the same fear and inability to deal with those emotions until I realized I wasn't 14. I had to keep reminding myself that I was an adult now, and that I was able to deal with my emotions. Each time I opened a box, I passed through all five stages of grief. Those emotions needed to be grieved, just as they had, when I had packed them.

Eighteen

MY
EXPERIENCE
WITH GRIEF

Age 27

"How could you?" I screamed, rage blowing out of me like a rocket. I felt betrayed, shocked and appalled. I felt sick with pain. My body ached as I stood there, glaring at my boyfriend. He had been admiring a beautiful, sexy woman on television when I walked into the room. I wanted to kill him like he was killing me. I wanted to hurt him like he was hurting me. I attacked him, with words that viciously slashed and degraded him. I accused him of cheating on me. I called him a betraying bastard who didn't care about anyone but himself. I called him a disgusting, pathetic person. Only disgusting, pathetic people had sexual fantasies about other women when involved in a relationship. I told him that he had a problem. Then I told him to go to hell. I ran out of the room and banged my fists on the wall, the banister and then my bed. I screamed and cried. I was in agony.

I cried and cried. I wanted to die. I asked God to take me to save me from this pain. I lay flat on my back, completely defenceless. My mouth was open wide as I cried out my hurt. I felt as though someone was pulling acid-like rope out of me — more and more kept coming as they pulled hand over hand. I just lay there, pinned down by the pain. I had no choice — the acid, the pain was coming out, there was no stopping it. The pain got worse. Suddenly, I felt as though it were someone else who was crying, not me. I could hear myself cry, but it wasn't me. It reminded me of the time I ripped the ligament in my right ankle away from the bone. The pain was so bad that, as I lay on the ground screaming, I wondered who was screaming.

Back in my room, I realized that it was me who was there on the bed crying and that I was feeling my pain as a baby. I was feeling betrayed, terrified, alone and abandoned, just as I must have as a baby. Where is everyone, I wondered fearfully? Is anyone there for me? Where am I? I want to die. I can't stand this.

Then, a strong loving part of me (the adult), embraced the little baby, like a parent would a child. I felt overwhelmed with love for that little baby. I understood the hurt and pain I had felt all those years ago. Now, finally, after having *rejected them for so many years, I had finally embraced the emotions I had felt as a defenceless baby. I was now whole.*

I had blamed my partner for betraying me, preparing to abandon me and inflicting so much excruciating pain on me. I had no idea that it was I who had the problem, I who owned the box, and I who needed to grieve. Now that I've gone through my grieving process, I know that my partner did nothing to warrant my accusations.

Months had passed since my dream about the warehouse of boxes. I had unpacked and grieved many before finding the box labelled: "Abandonment, birth — August 27, 1966." This box was at the back of the warehouse, the first one I'd stored away. Up until now, I had opened the boxes in reverse chronological order, from the present backwards. Although other boxes remained to be opened, that evening with my boyfriend, I headed straight for the first box.

The grieving process is an emotional journey with five stages. I see these stages symbolically as rooms in a house. The front door is the beginning of the process. Five rooms separate the front door from the back in this house of grief. The back door is the only way out. Each time I grieved, I entered by the front door, walked through each room, and exited through the back door. No other route could be taken. I had to fully experience the contents of each room before I could proceed to the next room, and then head out the back, otherwise, the grieving process would be incomplete and the box would still be there.

Although it took me 27 years to face the "abandonment" box, the box I feared the most, and to pass through all five stages of grief, I did it! I'm so grateful that I gained enough courage during my recovery to face that box and to feel it fully. Here's how I experienced the disintegration of that box and my own reintegration.

The first room was the "shock room." (Shock may occur when the mind, body or emotions are disturbed from a balanced state; change.) I was disturbed from a balanced state by being born. A change had occurred. I had lost my twin sister, my companion for nine months. No one was there to greet me when I was born into this cold, loud, bright world. I didn't know what had happened. I was terrified. I was unable to control or prevent my birth. I was utterly helpless. I entered the front door and stepped into the first room, the "shock room."

While in the "shock room," I wasn't aware of what was happening around me. I was stunned. This room allowed me time to synthesize the change that had occurred. The floor of this room consisted of one large cushion; it served to soften the blow. Then the shock began to wear off and I grew coherent enough to realize what had happened. I had been born. No one was there for me. I waited. Days passed, still no one. I was terrified. I panicked. I thought, I'm going to die. I hurt too much. I ran right into the next room, the "denial room," the second stage.

Terrified by what I had seen in the first room, I ran to the next room for safety. I slammed the door and pressed my back against it, gasping for breath. I was determined to get away from what was pursuing me. I immediately packed those horrible emotions into a box and put the box in a warehouse. (This was the first time I packed and stored a box.)

I packed it away with great speed because I wanted to get things back in balance, back to normal, as soon as possible. I desperately wanted things to be back the way they were. I wanted to be back in my warm, loving environment (in the womb) with my sister. I sat still, curled up in the corner of this room. Soon, the "denial room" began to work. I began to feel numb. I was so relieved to be feeling nothing. I knew I had to stay here as long as was necessary. Although I didn't like being confined to this room, the alternatives, returning to the first or progressing to the third, left me with no choice. I stayed. Each time I heard a noise from the first room, I panicked, as though the life-threatening pain would catch up with me at any minute. I lived in the second room, in denial, for much of my first 25 years of life, and especially during my eating disorder as I describe in Chapter 5, "My Escape." I lived in the fantasy room. The sign on the door read "pain not allowed."

The "denial room" was my place of safety, the place I could escape my pain and feel pleasure. As long as I was in the "denial room," I could deny anything. I had experienced "shock," packed a box, and denied all of it. I had built a defence system that nothing could penetrate. I could pretend about anything. Nothing happened until I decided it had. Nothing painful ever happened. I had locked myself into the "denial room," shutting out painful memories. When I began my recovery and wanted to recall my past, I couldn't do it. I could recall few events prior to age 10. For years, I stayed in this room, living in fantasy and eating. Until I was 27, I didn't care about whether I had been adopted, who my biological mother was, or the circumstances surrounding my adoption, or so I thought. The "denial room" was very effective.

Up to age 15, I only fantasized while in the "denial" room. Then, at 15, I experienced the intoxicating effects of binging. Food immediately became my priority and fantasies took a back seat, functioning as a supplement. The food felt so good and the pain was so bad, that before long, I had lost control of my eating. From 15 to 25, every time I felt the life-threatening pain from the first room, I binged. I had to, to stay safe, to flee the pain. I didn't see any other choices.

Many people have asked me why I didn't just stop binging or why I didn't just pick up the phone and call them when I felt the need to binge?

The truth was, I didn't stop to think, feel or do anything, from the moment I decided to binge until I was finished. I wouldn't stop. I was terrified. I was running like a terrified young girl from pain, pain I was convinced would kill me. I had to deny it. I had to run from it. I had to eat.

The third room was the "bargaining, searching and pining" room. For years, my goal was to never, ever feel the pain contained in the "abandonment box." However, years passed, and once I became a teenager, I tried to bargain with my pain. I stepped out of the "denial room" and into the "bargaining room." I bargained, telling myself if I lost weight I would be happy. I lost weight but my pain stayed with me. I lost more weight but the pain remained. I tried to lose weight for years, hoping that maybe one time, it would work, but it never did. I bargained to be a good girl, but the pain continued. I bargained to trade some of my enjoyment for less pain, but the pain persisted.

I restricted my intake of food, alcohol, parties, and everything else I enjoyed in the hopes that the pain would diminish, but it hung on tenaciously. I bargained that by reading and working hard, I would have less pain, but the pain did not leave me. My pain persisted, regardless of what I tried, and I tried just about every thing possible. Then, I tried to rationalize the pain away. I found myself constantly returning to the bargaining table. I felt like a failure every time my bargain didn't succeed, but I kept on bargaining.

I was still in the "bargaining room," and facing one failure after another. I was getting panicky. My chest was tightening, my heart was pounding and my body was trembling. My breath was shallow. I didn't know what to do, I didn't know where to turn. I felt like I was on a highway with a transport truck approaching me in my lane while another came up right behind me. I had no recourse. I couldn't believe that I could never be skinny enough. I couldn't believe that nothing worked. I searched for answers — my life depended on it. I thought and thought — there must be a way. I couldn't give up my last desperate attempt to escape.

My attention was scattered. I was doing five things at once. I was cleaning the washroom, working at the computer, washing the dishes, sorting family photographs, and talking on the phone. I could not and did not want to concentrate on just one thing. Then, I realized how I had been speaking to people. I was extremely jumpy and defensive. But, I was unable to slow down. I could not stop doing. I had to keep moving. I was scrambling, searching for a way to stay away from something. I was overwhelmed with panic. I lost control of my emotions and began to scream at my boyfriend at the time.

"Pining" meant acknowledging (pining down) the reality of the loss. Prior to my recovery, when I was in this section of the third room, I'd sprint back to the "denial" room. I went back and fourth from the "bargaining" room to the "denial" room. I had not yet progressed beyond the "bargaining room," until now. I ran upstairs into my room, closed the door, and flung myself onto my bed. I lay on my back with arms spread out to each side. I had succumbed to what felt like my demise. I entered the "depression room."

This room, the "depression room," was the one I most dreaded. By allowing myself to enter it, I felt that I was saying: "Go ahead and jump into shark infested waters, it's important to your recovery." As important as I knew this was, I was terrified. (There was a reason I had resisted it all those years.) This time, after having exhausted every bargain, search and plea, I knew that I had been defeated. My efforts to avoid this place, and having to experience this pain, had been futile. I had starved myself all those days, purged so many times, spent all those hours dwelling on my body size, lost weight, had the perfect slim body, spent most of my money on clothing and cosmetics, spent endless hours on my make-up and hair, and worn the most uncomfortable shoes. I had looked beautiful and been so slim, but nothing was enough — the men I dated were still attracted to other women. They could still abandon me. I finally had to admit failure. I gave up. I had no more energy to keep trying. I had been defeated. I didn't care what happened to me now. The door to the "depression room" was wide open and I had entered.

The "depression room" has three sections. The first section which was defeat and despair. Previously, when I had been in this room, I had run back into the denial room. This time, I didn't have the energy, or I would have. After stepping into this room, I immediately felt helpless. I had been defeated. I had lost the 27-year fight. I felt utter despair. I was overwhelmed with pain.

I knew those feelings well. I felt them before every binge. Again, I understood why I had to binge. Each time I got close to this pain I'd panic, struggle to get away from it and I would binge. I had to alleviate this horrendous pain as quickly as possible. I ate a lot. I realized that all I was trying to do was protect myself from pain that felt life-threatening. But, I had no more energy to protect myself. I was ready to die from the pain.

I cried and cried and cried. I didn't know what would become of me, I felt so totally devastated. I feared I couldn't possibly survive. Then I thought: "I don't want to be here anymore. Please just take me away. I don't care what happens to me!" I had completely surrendered — I had given up all control. I felt devastated by being alone in an incubator. I felt terrified of this world. I felt angry for having lost my warm, safe, loving environment (womb) with my sister. I felt the emotions of a baby. I really felt I was that baby, only days old. The feelings were overwhelming. I knew I would have died had I fully felt them then. Then I thought, God, why did you let this happen? What did I do wrong? I sank deeper into my pain. I felt needy and at the mercy of others. I wanted to die. I really wanted to die. How could people just leave me here? Where am I? Where is my sister? Why am I here alone? I have to get out of here. I hate this.

At this point, I was gasping for air. I was sobbing loudly, but I didn't care. It felt so good to cry. I wanted to scream, and did. I relived the very roots of my pain. Then I felt love and compassion for myself. I hugged myself. I told myself that I loved me. I began to feel safe, warm and comforted. I had taken myself back. I had embraced the hurt part of me that I had rejected long ago. I knew that I would never again reject myself. I was back together again, hurt and all. Then it ended. One hour after I had succumbed to my feelings of defeat and despair, it was all over. I had unleashed emotions in that hour that I had held inside me for 27 years. No one could have ever convinced me of the freedom I would feel. I had released an incredible burden. I didn't feel lonely or apart from anyone or anything. Instead I felt whole and loved. I stayed in bed for the rest of the night, and felt asleep, peacefully.

I woke up the next morning feeling lighter, happier and calmer then ever before. Later in the day however, to my surprise, I felt angry, and entered the next section of the "depression room." I didn't understand why. I knew I had just experienced a tremendous release of stored-up pain. I was unnerved by my feelings of anger. I stayed in this part of the room until I understood what was causing my anger. I asked myself what I was angry at. My immediate response was that I felt a lack of control. I was scared of the unknown. Living without the pain I carried was new. I didn't know how to handle peacefulness, happiness and calmness. I felt compassion for myself. Of course I felt out of control — I was. After this realization , I allowed myself to be angry. I went for a jog and then a long walk. I spent the rest of the day by myself, working and then reading a novel. I didn't want to inflict my anger on anyone and I wasn't about to deny it. I knew that this stage was temporary. It felt good to allow it.

While in this place, I had terrible thoughts about my biological mother and the hospital staff. I felt fury towards the people who had cared for me during my first days of life. Then I felt guilt (the third section of the "depression room") for being angry at them. It wasn't their fault and I'm sure they probably did their best to care for me. If they hadn't been there for me, I might have died. I knew that, at 16, my biological mother wouldn't have been equipped to raise my sister and me, so I couldn't fault her for not keeping us. I stayed in this section of the room for the rest of the day. I understood that my anger caused my guilt. I knew that my anger was natural and that I wasn't a bad person for having been angry. I stopped feeling guilty. I had accepted my experience at birth. I had entered the "acceptance room."

The fifth room was the "acceptance and restructuring" room. I had accepted my past. I had accepted that I felt abandoned, alone and terrified at birth. I no longer felt the need to change the past. I accepted it for what it was. In fact, my perspective of the past had changed. I felt at peace with it. It had happened, and now I was a better person for having experienced it. All desire to change what was, was gone. The need to lay blame was gone.

I felt forgiveness. I forgave my biological mother for giving me up for adoption. I forgave the hospital staff for not taking the place of my mother and providing the love, affection and nurturing I so desperately needed. Finally, I forgave myself for having disowned my emotions at birth. I forgave myself for having given up on myself at birth. I forgave myself for having been addicted to food. I forgave myself for having binged, purged and starved. I understood everything now. I felt compassion for myself and others. I understood that the choices had been made (i.e. adoption), were difficult for all of us. The past was the past, and it was okay.

I felt grateful for who I was and what I had received in my life thus far. I had come out of my depression with its narrow perspective and could see the world from a much more objective point of view. I looked forward to life. I was in a state of acceptance.

My life had been on hold, stagnant, for the years prior to my recovery. I felt freed by having finally traveled through the all the stages of grief and to grieve the box labelled "abandonment." During those stale years, I had been busy denying, bargaining and searching, but not living. Now, I could live. I was excited about beginning to restructure and reorganize my life. I began to restructure by cleaning up everything that I'd swept under the carpet and everything that I hadn't dealt with while I had been binging and purging.

I had survived the house of grief! I had shed many burdensome layers and was now free. I felt renewed and revitalized. My perspective had changed dramatically. Now, I could really see how I had been relating to the world around me. I had been very dependent on everyone, everyone but myself.

Nineteen

STEPPING
OUT OF
MY SYMBOLIC
WORLD

Age 28

I was intoxicated by his magical, powerful aura. He was so strong, so intelligent, so self-assured and so well-spoken. Everything would be perfect now that he was with me. Only moments earlier, I was frantically speeding through traffic in anticipation of having his strong arms around me. My heart was beating at a marathoner's pace. I felt a surge of energy from the adrenaline pumping through my body. Soon, I would be with him. I hit the accelerator. But, the closer I got, the more panicky I felt. I hadn't seen him for two days. For two days, I had sorely missed him. I had thought of little else. I longed for him. I needed him. I thought I'd die without him. I loved him. Now, we were together, and I hugged him, or rather held onto him, like a terrified child clutches a parent. With every breath, I drew in his masculinity, his strength. My panic subsided, for now. The tension of the previous two days flowed out of my muscles and disappeared. I felt happy. I felt alive. I felt relaxed and at peace. I could feel safe in the world, as long as he was with me.

This happened a week before I began to grieve the "abandonment box." We were just inside the door to his house. After I had hugged him long enough to let go of him, he closed the door and we made our way to the living room. I kept one hand on him the whole way. We snuggled together in front of the fireplace. The panic and emotion had settled.

The time passed quickly until it was midnight and time for me to go home. Our evening had been beautiful and loving. Although I didn't want to leave, I was exhausted and emotionally drained. I had gone from terror to panic to excitement and calmness, all within a mere 48 hours. Back at my apartment, I changed into my pyjamas, hopped into bed and pulled out my journal. I began to write:

I feel like half a person without him. I feel so vulnerable, so weak, so unprotected, so unsafe. I feel so afraid when he's not around. I hate when he goes away. He might never return. As long as he's here with me, I know I'll survive. I can't live without him. I can't stand the thought of living without him. I need him to depend on, to survive. Yet, I feel a constant, gnawing terror that I might have to experience life without him. Well, that just can't happen. I will never let that happen. But why is this? What makes me feel so scared? I wish I didn't feel so desperate for him, but I do. All I know is that I am scared that I will die if he isn't there to protect, love and take care of me.

A week later I opened the "abandonment box." It has now been two months since I completed that grieving. During the last two months I have been in the restructuring stage. I spent most of those 60 days reflecting on how I had been living. I came to terms with the knowledge that I had not been living in reality, but that I had been in the "denial room" for a long time.

A "symbol" is *something which stands for, represents or suggests another thing.*[1] I related to people and things as symbols. I attached meanings to them that weren't real. I attached feelings to them that weren't real. Their characteristics were symbolic, not real.

I hadn't wanted to feel reality. I hadn't felt safe at birth. I hadn't felt safe in the environment of the incubator. I hadn't felt safe with my emotions while in the incubator. So I decided not to have feelings about reality. Instead, I had feelings about symbols. Anyone or anything that made me feel loved, cared for, or eased the pain (of being alone in the incubator), symbolized safety and survival to me.

It was midnight and I was wide awake. One lamp lit my apartment dimly. I made some toast and herbal tea. I went into the living room, settled on the couch, and proceeded to eat my toast. I was deep in thought, barely aware that I was eating. I chewed each bite thoroughly, as though I were chewing on what I was trying to face. I didn't want to face what I knew to be true, that by grieving, I had come out of the denial room.

I could no longer take refuge in my safe, warm, exciting, exhilarating, symbolic fantasy world. As I stared into the darkness of the night, I realized that I had been living in my own world, in an unreal world, for a long time. I'd been having a 28-year waking dream. Feeling my grief had aroused me from that dream. Now, reality stared me in the face. I kept chewing. I chewed harder and harder until I was finished. I knew that my own dream was also finished. I felt like I was spinning in mid-air, with the rug yanked out from under me. I felt completely unhooked from everything. My roots had been severed. I was outside the "denial room," my oasis. It had been my home — my sanctuary — for a long, long time. I knew no other place.

Most mornings, I would wake up out of a dream. Waking meant the end of the dream and the characters and environment of the dream. When it

---

[1]Simon & Schuster, Inc., p 1356.

was a scary dream, I was grateful to wake up. When I had a wonderful, warm, exciting dream, I felt sad and disappointed upon waking. I would feel as though I had experienced a loss, as though something wonderful had ended. Whether the dream was bad or good, I lost the people and places in it. But, I could expect to lose those things, after all, it was only a dream. What I now grasped was the extent to which I had been living in a dream.

Awakening out of a 28-year dream brought with it enormous sadness. It felt as though I had lost everything, even though most of it hadn't been real. The people and places that had been part of my life, in my waking dream, had lost their symbolic meaning. The feelings that I had attached to each were obviously inaccurate. I could see that now. People had become human and places had become just places. My fantasy balloon had burst. Even though I had not been living in reality, my dream had been my reality. These losses were painful. Those symbols had been so real to me. I knew that I needed to grieve them.

I wanted to, but I refused to deny this reality. I wasn't about to go back into the "denial room" to live. (Just think, I could have denied that I had been living in denial all my life!) I knew that I was passing through the denial stage of grief. I also knew that it was only by facing it that I would get through it. This was my dream since I was a young girl.

I was safe, carefree and happy. I was loved by a tall, dark and handsome man. He was strong, smart and successful. I didn't have to worry about any-thing, especially being abandoned. He loved me more than life itself. We lived together in a beautiful home. My man protected our home and protected me — no one could hurt us. I felt very confident, never sad, lonely or scared. I knew that I could be successful at anything I tried. I could express myself in any way I wanted. I was loved. I was safe.

All I had ever wanted was to feel safe. I had wanted that feeling so badly. As long as I had a man in my life, I could keep my dream alive. I realized that for 28 years, I had surrounded myself with people and things that symbolized safety. I had been trying to live out my dream. I had tried to create my dream environment in real life. I related to everyone and every-thing as though they were part of my dream.

I finished my first cup of herbal tea and made another. It was now two in the morning and I wasn't the least bit sleepy. Though I felt pro-found sadness, I also felt great compassion for myself. I understood why I had done so many of the things I had. I was beginning to understand how I had been relating to men and to food.

Men were symbols of safety, security and survival. Intelligence, con-fidence, physical and emotional strength, career success and financial sta-bility were all traits linked to this and I was attracted to men who had those characteristics. I was attracted to men could make me feel safe and take me away from pain. I was attracted to what a man symbolized, not who he was as a person.

I reread the journal entry I made the night I raced to see my man. I shook my head as I realized that I had been living on an emotional roller-coaster. I had driven at breakneck speed that night, desperate for the safety of his arms. I realized that I had panicked that same way many times before, with other men. I had never questioned it. In fact, I used to think that being distraught and practically unable to live while away from my partner somehow proved my deep and abiding love for him. This logic now amazed me.

I now knew that it wasn't love that made me spend days doing nothing but longing for a man, focusing on nothing but him. I had put my life on hold again, just as I had so many times before, because I had felt so unsafe and terrified while apart.

I believed I had to depend on a man to support me. I was convinced I wasn't capable of earning a good income and being successful in my own right. No, I needed a successful, financially viable man to take care of me. A successful, financially viable man symbolized my survival. I had starved myself so as to be attractive enough to make a man want me, love me, take care of me, keep me safe and stay with me forever. I was sure that this was my only chance for a safe, happy and pain-free life and I was willing to do whatever it took to keep a man with me. When I told someone that I loved him, I was really telling him that I felt safe and secure with him. I confused safety for love. I really had no idea what love was. I didn't love him, I needed him.

I needed a man to avoid feeling the pain of losing my mother. It was no accident that I got my first boyfriend at age seven, right after my mother left. I replaced my mom with a boy. I always had a boyfriend. Each time a relationship ended, I thought I'd die, even when I didn't care that much about him. Each of my boyfriends rescued me from the painful loss of my mother.

Food was a symbol. Food was my best friend. Food was my companion. Food had stuck with me throughout my life, it was always there to comfort me. Food was powerful. When I was a baby and most vulnerable, I was at the mercy of others for food. As a baby just prior to eating...

I lay in my crib. I was starving. I felt miserable. I felt angry. I felt awful. Then, food came, and took all that hurt away. I felt centred. I felt better. I felt enjoyment. I felt relieved. I felt awed by what this stuff (food) could do. I felt safe. I felt loved. I felt rescued. I knew that I would survive.

Food could make me feel so many things. I really did need food to survive, it was not just symbolic. I learned the power of food early. I had remembered all the feelings I had as a baby. During my 10-year eating disorder, so many years later, I felt those same feeling at full volume. I wanted to feel safe and loved. Food symbolized safety, survival and love. (Again, I had confused feeling safe with being loved.) Food symbolized emotion. I lost all awareness that it was a physical substance.

When I was in the crib, hungry, I felt unsafe and afraid, fearing for my survival. Once I was fed, my fear disappeared. As an adult, when my partner was not with me, I felt unsafe and afraid, fearing for my survival. Once I fed myself, my fear disappeared. The only problem was that my relief from fear was only temporary. I had to keep eating, and eating a lot. I overate and kept the food down. When I kept down the food, I kept down the feelings of safety, love and survival.

Then, food became my enemy when I gained weight. I felt betrayed. I had so completely trusted my loyal, loving and dependable companion. Gaining weight devastated me — I didn't know where to turn. By this point, I was feeling betrayed by men, my mother, my family — everyone and everything — and now food. So I purged, for the first time. I felt so good, as though I was telling food that I didn't need it, that I could dispose of it whenever I wanted. Nevertheless, I knew that I did need food. I grew to hate that need. I hated to need anything, but food was my only solace. Still, I had to show it who was boss, who was in control. I kept my food down as infrequently as possible, only when I was too tired to purge, or too needy for love.

I went to bed. It was now three o'clock and I was sleepy and happy. I knew how I had been living and why. I could recall times of shock, disappointment and fear when a man became human. I remember feeling let down that he was not as strong, intelligent and confident as I thought he was. He was actually human, just like me. I hadn't wanted him to be human. I had wanted to be taken care of. I had wanted to be safe. I had wondered who was going to take care of me. Now I knew why I would not allow my partner to be human. I knew it was time to relate to him as a human being; not a symbol. I turned out my light and went to sleep.

A few months later, after having experienced the depression stage of grieving the loss of many symbols, I was once again restructuring my life. I was ready to begin living outside the "denial room," and in reality. I was about to let go of my need to control, my need to control my partner, food and my pain.

```
*********
Twenty
*********
```

MY
SPIRIT
WORLD

Age 27-29

I was in the shower. I picked up the soap and began to wash. My mind was elsewhere, fretting about the ridiculous phone call I had just received. Suddenly, I felt a strong and loving presence. I looked around me and saw nothing. Then I had a magnificent vision of another world. I could picture this world, a beautiful and loving spirit world. In this world, spirits moved by floating; they were made of energy. I knit my brows and questioned my sanity. The next moment, my doubt disappeared and my vision returned. The vision was very real. The spirit world did exist. I had not lost a grip on my sanity. Its presence was overpoweringly warm and beautiful.

No words were spoken. No sounds were heard. It was all sensations — of a loving, peaceful energy. I immediately discerned that this world existed beyond the physical level and I could feel a deep connection with it. I understood that the physical world (the earth) and this spirit world, were to function as one. I, and the spirits of this world, were to function as one. I understood where I came from, where to take my direction from and who to follow. I understood that my true home was the spirit world. I understood that my guides for my time on earth were spirits. I understood the meaning of spirituality.

That day, one year after I had begun my recovery, I finally understood about my attraction to nature, to goodness and to love. Everything I had longed for, for so many years, made up the spirit world. Even though my vision of it lasted for only minutes, it was all I needed. I knew that world; it was as familiar as a childhood home and I felt very connected to it. I felt so excited. From that moment, I knew (not just thought) that a spirit world existed.

I had been living as though I were separate from the spirit world. I had been living as though only physical and mental worlds existed. I had been focused on my body size and consumed by my thoughts. I had been disconnected from the true source of life — a spiritual life. I now believe that I am a spiritual being having a human experience. I believe that my

home is in the spiritual world. I believe that I had been trying to reconnect with the spirit world for 27 years. Now I know I am connected.

I had been trying to connect with the spiritual world through food,
men, and fantasy. I had been using these to try to recreate all the familiar,
spiritual feelings. I longed to connect more than anything in this world.
But it wasn't in this world where I would find the means to connect.
Nothing physical would take me there. Nothing mental either. I was busy
for 27 years trying to connect using all the wrong things. I was connected
already. I just had a 27-year memory lapse. Now I remember. I was about
to enter the world I had so long ago forgotten. I was about to begin a
relationship between my spiritual self and the spirits of the spiritual world.

Getting to the point where I felt comfortable relating to the spirit
world didn't happen overnight. After experiencing the euphoria of envi-
sioning my spiritual home, I returned to the real world. What with every-
day mundane tasks, the violence and greed of this world, and continuing
my painful recovery, I had difficulty holding onto my vision. Doubts began
to seep in. My moods tempered the love and excitement I had felt. If a
world of so much love existed, why didn't I feel happier? Yet, I held onto
my vision. I knew it was true. I could have dismissed it by chalking it up
to a figment of my overactive imagination. Yet, I knew otherwise. If I were
to have dismissed it, I would have missed yet another opportunity to
experience my spirituality.

Before I began my recovery, I had been closed, unwilling to believe
that anything spiritual, loving or positive existed in this world. In fact, I
thought that people who believed in and practised religion were weak
and lacking in control and drive. Besides, I was angry at everyone because
I had been abandoned at birth. I was not about to open my heart and
place my faith in something, just to be abandoned again. No way!

Unfortunately, all those years that I had rejected the existence of spirituality, I had missed receiving the help, love and support from that world.
I believe that messages are passed from the spirit world to earth through
people, places and things. I had missed many words of wisdom from
people, and many meanings from coincidental circumstances. While I
felt detached from that world, it had been trying to communicate with
me all along and I had not been able to receive it. I had the radio cranked
up to the loudest volume most of the time. I could barely hear my own
friends speak. For years, my most commonly used word was "pardon?" I
had been extremely closed-minded about anything beyond my control. I
wasn't the easiest person to communicate with.

Then I began my recovery. During the first year, I could not write off
many unusual phenomena. I saw things I had not seen before. I heard
things I had not heard before. Before I knew it, I had begun to appreciate

these coincidences. In fact, I had begun to anticipate them. I looked forward to experiencing a coincidence even while a part of me had remained sceptical. After one year, I had my vision in the shower. Then, I understood where the coincidences came from.

As I have described, throughout my recovery, I received help just when I needed it. I was given just the right book to read when I needed an answer. I bumped into just the right person when I needed a connection for a job. I had just the right road sign that allowed me to proceed in my travels. I had just the right distraction to miss the car that had run the red light in front of me. So many coincidences! Help and answers had been provided just when I needed them. Unfortunately, although I appreciated the coincidences at the time, minutes later, I would forget them.

I knew that a spirit was always looking out for me — I could feel it. I would often joke to my close friend that whoever was protecting me sure had their hands full! I wished I could say I always appreciated the help, but I didn't. Every now and then, absorbed in my own challenges, a warm gesture from a stranger would remind me of my spirit. One afternoon, I read an article in a magazine that described how Angels communicate to humans. One example was the presence of a feather out of nowhere. An hour later I went into the den and stood awestruck as I watched a feather fall from the ceiling and land on my usual spot on the couch. I felt a rush of warmth, love and gratefulness. I looked up and said thank you. Some days I felt awe and love, other days, I would not stop to appreciate those communications. Whether or not I stopped, a spirit was always with me.

By now, two years into recovery, I understood more about spirits and the spirit world. Some people call those spirits God, Buddha, Zen, Angels, etc. I knew that I had a guardian Angel who was always with me. I understood that my Angel was a part of God, and worked on His behalf. My relationship with my spirit and the spiritual world is a personal, one-on-one relationship.

Even though I had a guardian Angel who was always with me, I couldn't help being scared sometimes. I'd feel weak for being afraid after all I had been shown. (One year later, I understood that being fearless was impossible until I had fully grieved.) At this point in my recovery, I still felt unlovable, untrustworthy and incapable. I feared that if a spirit asked something of me, I would let it down. I just didn't know enough about myself and the spirit world yet. Our relationship was still growing; it was in the early stages.

I prayed almost every morning. On mornings when I felt fearful, I would say the "Lord's Prayer," so quickly that even the most astute of listeners would never have understood. Many of my prayers were brief.

Sometimes, I would pray for things and then say to myself: "Well that will never come true." When it didn't, I would say: "See, there is no such thing as a spirit. I am crazy. If there is a spirit, then I don't deserve what I asked for." Then I would zip off to wherever I was headed that day, without the slightest feeling of trust, faith or love.

Other mornings, I would pray to the spirit and feel safe and loving. Sometimes those feelings lasted all day. Other days, noon would come and all would be lost. Then I would feel very disappointed with myself for not trusting. After all, I had had the vision in the shower. I thought that I should be able to wake up every morning feeling love and happiness. I thought that I should have left my fear behind. Not so. Trust, excitement and love often took a back seat to my fear. There would be many days without trust or love. Though my faith and trust were often momentary, they did exist, and were growing.

Outside of coincidences, I received communications from the spirits primarily through my feelings. I could sense them, much like I had in the shower, yet less intensely. Sometimes I would wonder what choice to make. At those time, my sixth sense, which is my spiritual sense, and my gut reaction would lead me to make the right choice, a spiritual choice. So now the communication between me and the spiritual world was via prayer, feelings and coincidences. I kept on praying, feeling and appreciating the coincidences.

Despite my fear, I pressed on in my recovery. I had been recording my dreams each morning since the beginning of my recovery. Nothing in particular had prompted me to record them, I just felt the need to. (Another feeling, a communication from the spirit world that I act on.) I intuitively knew that dreams were very important. But I would often find the meaning of my recorded dreams hard to understand. So I bought books on dream interpretation. I learned that dreams were a communication from the unconscious to the conscious. I knew that I always felt different after a dream, changed in some way. My dreams were like information-filled movies. They showed me how I was feeling, the emotions I was repressing, the people who had affected me and what direction my life needed to take. I learned so many things because I paid attention to my dreams. My relationship with myself and my spirit world grew close and strong because I paid attention to them.

Even though I read lots of books on dreams, I was far from an expert. Sometimes I didn't have a clue what they meant. But that didn't matter. Sometimes I would understand my dream only weeks after having bumped into the person or hearing a sound that had been in my dream. I did know, however, that my dreams were messages from the spiritual world.

I was in a house, Olga's house, a three-story home. I was trying to teach an aerobics class but couldn't find an aerobics cassette tape. I couldn't begin the class without the right music. When I found one, I only played one song before the tape jammed. I felt so disappointed for having to stop the class. As much as I tried, I could not replay the tape. Then I was in another room. This room was across the hall. The room was filled with mostly women and a few men, about 30 people all-told. These people were feeling grateful. I had been talking to them about my experience of overcoming my eating disorder. I could feel their feelings. They didn't feel alone anymore. When I was finished my talk, some of them came to me to ask specific questions. I talked to each person privately. I could feel that these people were about to begin their recovery. They desperately wanted to know how to begin. I told them about how I had recovered.

When I had that dream, I had been managing a business that provided aerobic classes. I had been teaching three classes a day and had little time to write or give seminars on my recovery. I dreamed that the aerobic classes were over (the tape jammed), and that people wanted to hear about my recovery. "Olga" means "holy"; I was in a "holy house," a home. Three weeks later, I sprained my ankle severely. My ability to teach aerobics came to an abrupt stop. Two days after my injury, I began writing this book on a full-time basis. I wrote from an office in my three-story home. Although I had written much of the book already, I hadn't had time to focus on it. Writing between teaching aerobic classes and running a business had been challenging. Now I had time. I wrote all day, every day, for the next six months. My dream had taken form. I knew just what to do — I had to write.

Many of my dreams revealed what I needed to do in life. Believing that dreams are one way spirits can communicate with me, I took the meanings of my dreams very seriously. When I'm asleep, my defences are down and I'm more receptive to messages. I never downplay a dream. They are precious to me.

I felt close to the spiritual world when I went for walks. To me, nature exuded spiritual energy. When my mind was quieted or freed from distracting thoughts, I could communicate with the spiritual world. Just breathing was like breathing in spirit. I would inhale spirit and exhale fear. Meditation, for me, was sitting and relaxing, while feeling myself breathe. I would sit in the den in peace and privacy, listening to my breathing. In this way, I could separate from my thoughts. I could understand what was happening inside me. I would let myself think whatever thoughts I wanted. It took me three years to be fearless enough to meditate in this way. By slowing my mind and my body, I began to understand many things that were bothering me. When thoughts came up, I would picture them as though they were each inside a bubble. Sitting on the shore of a river, I would watch the bubbles flowed down with the current. Sometimes I would converse with my thoughts.

I was breathing when a bubble passed that contained a fearful thought. The fear was that I wouldn't be successful in taking care of myself. The old fear message had shown itself, as some of my fears did when I let them surface. I asked the fear what it meant. It said that I didn't have the brains, drive or strength to be able to have a career and earn an income that would sustain me. I said, really? Have I never been able to earn an income? My fear said, well yes… but… I said: Okay I realize that I'm unsure about my future in business. But I 'll try to do my best to do what I can right now. I will strive to become more successful.

That fear was gone now. It flowed down the river. Had I not faced the fear, I might have spent the entire day panicking about my future. Now I could do something about it. I faced a few other fears like that one that day. I reasoned with many of my fears, worries, doubts in that way, for the second two years of my recovery. I tried not to suppress the messages in the bubbles. Sometimes I was scared to face them and other times I wasn't. I faced them on my own time. I wanted to face them because I knew that otherwise I would be consumed by them. I knew that they usurped much of my energy. When I was consumed by them, I couldn't communicate with the spirit world. My relationship with the spirit world was my priority.

I read books on the Near Death Experience (NDE) and gained a deeper and more inspiring understanding of the spiritual world. I am grateful to those authors for writing about their experiences. I gained so much strength for my own spiritual life from reading those stories. I realized that there are many sceptical people who don't believe in the reality of NDEs. I also realize that an NDE cannot be proven scientifically, but that is irrelevant to me. I respect the position of those who don't believe, but I do.

Every day I grew closer to spirits and the spiritual world. My faith took what seemed like eternity to grow. For the next two years, I recorded my dreams, I prayed and faced the messages in the bubbles. Some days, I communicated and other days, I didn't. Some days I received answers, other days I didn't. When I felt apart from the spirit world, it was because I had closed the door. All I ever had to do was look up and say hello. I would smile. A spirit was always with me. I knew that one day I would have a relationship with my own spirit and the spiritual world that included trust, love and faith. That day has arrived.

Twenty-One

I WAS
LEARNING
ABOUT ME

Age 29

My friend had barely heard a word I said all morning. I felt left out of his world. Since I had grieved the abandonment box, the weight of the world had lifted, but I also felt strangely unhinged. The pain I had dragged around with me for many years was gone. It had been like an anchor, weighing me down. Now, I felt as though I were in the middle of a river with neither shore in sight. For the last two months, I had been resting from the pain of recovery. I was floating in the middle of the river, holding onto a life-preserver. My friend's support was the one thing that had remained constant, and now I felt detached from him too. I didn't feel panicky or afraid, just very uneasy.

I went to the den to be alone. I sat on the couch and began to converse with my feelings. I was trying to identify the source of my uneasiness. I did what I usually did to face my thoughts and emotions. I closed my eyes and pictured myself standing beside a river. I watched the bubbles flow by. I asked myself the question: "What's causing your uneasiness?" "Being apart from my friend," I replied. "What would happen if you were apart from him?" I pressed on. "I don't know. I used to think that I couldn't survive without him, but now I know that message is false." "Are you certain that you no longer need him to survive?" "Yes," I responded, "I'm certain I could survive without him, but I don't want to. This isn't about my survival." "Okay then, what is it about?" "I'm feeling unhooked. Nothing is familiar anymore. Everything is new. My pain is gone and I'm grateful, yet it was so familiar. It was like an old friend, a painful one, but a known quantity. Now that it's gone, I have no direction or focus. My friend gives that to me. Now I realize that it's time to take direction from me."

I sat in silence for a moment. I had my answer. I was apprehensive about letting go of my friend as my only source of support. At once, I knew that I was in a period of great change. I looked up to the ceiling and asked my guardian Angel: "Why is this change so hard for me? This is what I've always wanted and worked so hard for. Why am I resisting?" Then I knew why. This change was really big. I had never actually relied on myself before. As uneasy and uncomfortable *as I was, I was ready to make the transition. I took a deep breath in preparation to step out of this in-between stage, from relying on others to relying on me. I looked up and asked my Angel to help me make this transition. I felt a warmth flood all over my body. I felt a surge of strength and reassurance. I knew I would be okay. My heart was dancing. I no longer felt angry, abandoned or alone. I wasn't alone — I had me.*

I had chosen to live my own life. I stopped spending my precious time and energy worrying about what everyone else was thinking and doing and began to focus on me. I was ready to get to know me. Changing that focus seemed like a huge leap from one mountain to the next. Yet when I made the choice, it was like one regular step. There was no big drop between mountains and no grave consequences to my survival. I suppose that I was more ready that I realized. I had been in recovery for more than three years.

Everything was unfamiliar. I was in the middle of a river, having swum from a past shore, on my way to a future shore. I didn't know what I would find on the unfamiliar, unknown shore. I could have gone back to the familiar shore. But, no way! I could never go back to an unreal, unhealthy and unrewarding life. I chose to find myself, regardless of the consequences. I swam on and reached the other side.

I was experiencing a major turning point in my recovery. Previously, my recovery was about letting go and grieving. I had been swimming away from things, leaving my past behind. I no longer carried the old pain and hurt. Now it was time for me to take back important parts of me, parts that I had rejected long ago. I let go of the life preserver and began to swim toward my future, myself.

As ready as I was, I still felt uneasy about facing me. What if I don't like myself? What if I don't have any good qualities or skills? Speculation and worry flooded my head. I took a deep breath. I knew those worries were natural. After all, I was beginning something incredibly different, something I had perceived as the scariest thing I could ever do — face myself.

I reminded myself that I was about to build a relationship with a person I barely knew. I needed to know what tools I had been born with. I needed to know what I had to work with. I needed to see what I had to offer the world. I wanted to know how I could function in the world as me. I felt as though I was about to meet someone new. I had hopes, and anxieties, that this relationship with myself would work. (Beginning a relationship with another person was much easier. I could walk away from them if I didn't like them. I can't walk away from me. I had no way out.)

I began to pace. I was nervous about getting to know myself. After minutes of useless pacing, I asked myself if pacing would make me a better, more likable person. Am I not the person who is standing here right now? If I sit down, will that soften having to face me? No, but by facing me now, I will know who I am. That will make a difference. I knew that putting off facing me wouldn't help me become me. I realized that I didn't have to like everything about myself. I also realized that I might like parts of me, I could be surprised. Either way, I would deal with the likes and dislikes as they emerged. I decided to take it one step at a time. I didn't want to reject me any longer. I wanted to live as me.

I got into my car and set out for a hillside close to where I lived. Every time I was about to get closer to myself, I went to nature. Although my Guardian Angel was always with me, I felt an even greater strength when I was in nature. I arrived at my wondrous destination. I followed the road's curves, heights and valleys. Both sides of the road were sculptured with big, beautiful trees that radiated an unbelievably loving, spiritual presence. I felt so welcomed each time I visited. I took a deep breath, drawing in that beautiful, loving life-filled energy. I came to a fork in the road and veered to the right. I pulled into a park surrounding a small lake. I got out of my car and walked down to the shore. I looked straight down into the water and it mirrored my reflection. The sounds of nature played like a might and captivating symphony. I looked up to the sky and I knew that with the help of my Guardian Angel and the magnificent strength and love of nature, I would learn about me. I would learn with my eyes only, without the eyes of society. I began with the basics. I had a brain. I had a body. I had a spirit.

I HAD A BRAIN. My brain functioned like everybody else's. It had electrons, nerve impulses, neuro-transmitters and all its various centres. I had thoughts and ideas. I had theories and understandings. I had opinions. I knew that I had the technology, the brain. Everything was in working order.

I had thoughts, ideas and opinions. (My ideas were often different than those of other people.) I had a voice and could articulate them. I had been quiet for so long. I could speak about what I thought, not what someone else thought. I had my own words. No one could say my words were right or wrong; they were mine. I was the only person who could offer my thoughts, ideas and opinions.

I could read and write. Yes, I did have difficulty understanding certain things. I often had to work hard to understand what I had read. I definitely had to work hard to learn how to write. But I knew that I had a brain that functioned. Since I hadn't exercised it, I had to apply my best efforts to learn. (I felt like I was blowing the cobwebs out.) I wasn't afraid though, because I knew I had a good, working brain.

I drove home. As usual, I had received so much insight from nature. I felt energized and even more motivated to be me.

A few days later, I was standing in front of the mirror. It was early morning and I was fresh out of the shower. I was feeling happy. I felt smart, and that alone made me feel stronger. I felt like I could cope. I briefly retraced my steps to this point. I had come a long way in just the last three or so years. I felt so much joy and pain. I felt like I was living a new life. I had left so much behind. I really felt good about myself that morning. For the first time, I liked the person in the mirror.

Then I looked at my legs. For 29 years, every time I looked in the mirror, my eyes went directly to my legs, and my face puckered in disgust. This time, I thought: Gee, my legs really don't look that bad! I indulged myself by actually admiring my legs — for the first time! I thought: "Hey, I like them! They're not that bad, maybe they're even nice." For the next few minutes, I vacillated from: "Are they really okay?" to "They're nice!" I changed angles, offering myself a side view. I liked the side view even better. I tried the other side, still okay. I couldn't help but smile. I felt myself smile from inside. I felt happy. I liked my legs. They were okay! They were my legs!

I HAD A BODY. I had blond hair, green eyes, stood 5'8 3/4", weighed 127 pounds, had muscular legs and a petite bust. I had a slim waist and hips. I was active in many sports. I had good hand-eye coordination. I had good endurance and strength. I had lived in this body for 29 years and hadn't appreciated any of those characteristics. I had always wanted to be different — different was better.

I had red highlights in my blond hair, especially if I had been in the sun. I wore pink to fight against that. I had always wanted blue eyes, appreciating everyone's eyes but mine. I had wanted a larger bust and much smaller legs. I wanted to be better in every sport. I had not appreciated that I was quite good in some. Overall, I hadn't appreciated what I had. I always wanted to be one step better. I didn't even know what better was. I had always wanted to a new and improved version of me — but not any more.

A few mornings later, I stood in front of the mirror again. My legs had been okay, so maybe, just maybe, I would try again. I looked at my bust. So often, I would press my arms up against each side of them to make them look bigger. Now I saw my breasts as they really were. They were small. That was a fact, as much as I resisted accepting it. What I had failed to notice before was that they were firm and in proportion. I actually liked them. Then I realized that I had never done a breast exam. I wouldn't touch them before. I had never touched them. For twenty-plus years they had been on my body, but I had never touched them! I couldn't believe it! So I did. I touched them and they felt nice. I didn't race from the room screaming in terror. Actually, they felt larger than they looked. I was thrilled. I stood tall, with my stomach in and chest out. I felt proud of my bust. I felt like a kid with a new toy. I had just received me.

I was no longer fighting what nature had given me. I was beginning to appreciate my physical appearance. This was the way I looked , so I figured, why not work with it? I liked my legs. I liked my reddish-blonde hair and green eyes. I wore clothes that enhanced my body shape. I stopped trying to wear what everyone else was wearing. I had larger legs than most woman so most skirts looked terrible on me. I stopped trying to lose weight on my legs to wear those skirts; I began to wear skirts that flattered me. Shopping became fun. I began to look positively at the shopping experience. So many clothes looked awful on me. So I just kept trying things on. As long as I persevered, I would find something that fit well. As well, instead of fretting about my tough-to-fit shape, I told myself that my body shape was unique. And it was. Very few manufacturers cut clothes to fit me. How much more unique can a person get?

I wanted to take care of my body. I didn't want to starve it any longer. I wanted to nourish it with protein, carbohydrates, vitamins and minerals. I got eight hours of sleep every night and drank 10 glasses of water a day. I ate only when I was hungry and only good, nutritious foods. I cared about my body. I had chosen to nurture it. My body was the temple of my spirit.

I HAD A SPIRIT. I had feelings. I had emotions. I had strength. I had motivation. I had intuition. I had creativity. I had all of those things, and at the core of it all was love. My spirit was love, my heart was love. My spirit was the most important part of me. I had a brain so I could learn things and I had a body so I could go places. But, I was spirit above all else.

As I described in the last chapter, I had gained a faith in God, Angels and my Guardian Angel. My spirit is what communicates to the spirit world. I receive communication from the spirit world through my feelings. My own spirit communicates to me, my brain and body, through my feelings. I feel my spirit when I feel happy, sad, angry, joy, etc. No one can tell me not to cry, not to overreact, or not to be so sensitive. I felt what I felt. I felt my spirit. My spirit was never wrong. I was thrilled that I was feeling! Finally, after years of not feeling, I was, and it was okay, more than okay, it was wonderful. I cried when I wanted to and laughed when I wanted to. I no longer felt ashamed. I knew that it took courage to feel. It didn't take courage to deny. I wondered why a person who denied their feelings was considered a martyr.

I knew more about myself than ever before. I had qualities, skills and talents that were just waiting to be exercised. I had a brain, a body and a spirit. I felt like an artist ready with paint brushes, paints and canvas. Now, I faced a new challenge — to maintain my centredness amid negative external influences. I was about to paint, to be me in this world. I was ready.

Twenty-Two

I DEVELOPED
A BOUNDARY

Age 29

O ne afternoon, I was walking down the street on my way to meet my girlfriend for lunch. I was wearing shorts and a tank top, nothing revealing, just something casual and cool. This spring day was beautiful and warm and I was feeling particularly good. It was so great to be outside again. The winter had been long and cold, with a record snowfall. As I walked along the sidewalk of this busy street, I could feel many eyes on me, mostly men's. My first reaction was to make sure that I was walking okay and that I looked okay. Then, I said to myself: "Hey wait a minute, I'm going to walk the way I walk." But the very next thoughts were: "What will happen if I don't make sure I walk okay? Will people be disgusted? Will they reject me?" The thoughts arrived so fast I couldn't believe it.

I chose to respond to my thoughts this way: "I understand that I'm shy about revealing who I am. I understand that it's risky to be me and perhaps have other people reject me. But I am me and I'm going to honour myself and take the chance that I'll be rejected. What does rejection mean to me now, anyway? How will being rejected by someone affect my life? It won't. I'm no longer so dependent on the opinions of others. Besides, the people on this street are strangers! I don't even know them."

So, I made a decision. I said to myself: "I know it feels weird, but I'm going to walk the way I walk. I am going to show myself who really matters. Though I had been walking all that time, I stood even straighter, held my head high, and kept walking. People kept looking, some people frowned, others smiled. For the first time, their reaction to me was not important to me. I felt confident. I knew who I was. I was smart. I was pretty. I had feelings.I was a kind person. I was honest. I had come full circle. I was being me, regardless of how the people around reacted to me. I was happy to be me — finally.

When I got to the restaurant, my girlfriend hadn't arrived yet. Another friend came over to say hello. He sat down and proceeded to tell me that my outfit was "interesting"(not a compliment), and my choice of words "improper." I became upset. Then, he quietly told me to "relax." Now, I was downright mad.

I couldn't believe it. Moments earlier, I had been so happy and proud to be who I was. All of that centredness left me. I regrouped. I said to him: "I like my outfit. My choice of words is proper. And I'm not going to 'relax' and listen to you any longer." I got up and asked for another table. I sat down and shook my head. I was stunned by his words and by what had just happened. I hadn't expected my "friend" to relate to me in that way. He was normally so gracious.

I was sitting quietly when my girlfriend finally arrived. Needless to say, I was happy and relieved to see her. Her first words were about how much she loved my outfit! I told her about my earlier conversation, or rather, confrontation. My graphic and animated description got us both laughing. It felt so good to put that scenario in a humorous context, in its proper perspective. Previously, I might have spent hours being bothered by his words. My girlfriend couldn't believe that my friend didn't like my outfit, and that he had told me to relax. We were both amazed at his perception of me, and how it was so different from ours. I knew his words had nothing to do with me. I knew who I was.

Life. Was it ever tough sometimes. I had come so far in my recovery, then boom! A few harsh words from a friend were all it took to crack my foundation. It seemed as though my recovery went right out the window. Well, it wasn't quite that extreme, but it sure felt like it. However, for the few minutes I was listening to my friend, I lost touch of myself. I wished I could just be myself, unaffected by what others said or did. Unfortunately, it wasn't that simple —people did matter to me. I loved having people in my life. Now, I would learn about how to be me and maintain my composure and centredness, while relating to others.

I could have written an entire book describing how I developed this protection, how I acquired my boundary and how I learned how to recognize the signs of a potential boundary violation. I feel very strongly about protecting people who don't have boundaries, and can't protect themselves. When I sat down to write this chapter, I starting describing all the ways I learned to build and use my boundary and ended up with 15 pages. I decided to concentrate on the most important ways.

I feel very strongly about boundary violations because, for many years, I allowed people to say things to me that hurt. I allowed people to do things that hurt. And I said nothing, but cried inside. This chapter isn't about those violations — they are over. What is important is how I live today, and how I protect myself right now. I honour, protect, love and nurture myself the best way I can today. By having a boundary, I can function more easily in a world where so many people hurt others. I wish with all my heart that people would stop hurting each other. I feel so protective of myself now and I exercise that protection. I wish everyone else could as well. Very few people hurt me now.

By this point in my recovery, I had attained a clear sense of who I was. I knew how I felt and what I wanted in life. Although I was far from perfect, I accepted the person who lived in my skin and liked her. I would never have believed that I would ever get to this point. I never thought it was possible to wake up in the morning and smile, simply because I'm me. I never thought that I'd be excited to be myself and happy to be alive. Some days I felt angry and other days I felt sad. But every day, I was feeling, and feeling very grateful to be me.

I had acknowledged my mind, body and spirit. I knew what I was made of. I knew what was inside me and understood my thoughts and feelings. I knew my exterior, my body. I vibrated with my mind and spirit, within my body. My body gave me five senses. Now I had gained a sixth sense — I had developed a boundary.

My boundary was an invisible energy that surrounded my body. My energy field (my sixth sense) sensed my surroundings. This energy field was an aura that radiated energy like a bulb radiates light. My boundary sensed the outside world like a natural form of protection. My boundary protected me from unwanted intrusion. My boundary protected my mind, body and spirit. No one could intrude unless I allowed them to.

I finally felt safe in my own skin. I had gained a sense of myself. I didn't have to be overly influenced by others. Somebody might try to tell me what I thought, but I could disagree, I knew what I thought. Somebody could tell me I needed to lose weight, but I knew I didn't. Somebody could tell me that I couldn't be happy about something, but I knew what I felt.

Feeling came much more naturally now. The habit of denying my feelings was gone, it had just slipped away without my awareness. Now, I was a friend to myself and I could feel my own presence. For years, I lived in my body, but never realized it. Now I was good company to myself. Previously, when I spent time alone, I had felt very lonely. Yet, I was vibrating in there the whole time. I had been so focused on the outside world that I didn't even realize that someone lived inside my skin. But, someone did, and I vowed never to turn away from her again.

Acquiring a boundary was connected to feeling my emotions. My boundary is like a sixth sense. It's instinctual. Had I been able to think a boundary into existence, I would have. But my boundary did not grow from thought. If it had, I would have always had one. I came to feel myself in my skin and care about me after four years of recovering, of feeling. I used to think: "I don't have to allow that person to talk to me in that condescending way." But then, when I allowed them to, and reacted with hurt, I thought I somehow must be to blame for it, that I should have prevented it. I would say to myself: "You didn't have to let them get to you."

I didn't actually realize when a person had crossed my boundary until I was well into my recovery. (I use the word cross to describe a boundary intrusion. My boundary is a circle around me and a person who got to me had crossed over that circle into me.) Although my boundary had always existed, I couldn't feel it. I had been in the "denial room" and had felt nothing. It was like my foot was paralyzed and I couldn't feel anything when a person stepped on it, I could only watch. I couldn't sense when someone was approaching my boundary. I didn't know where it was until I began to feel. Feeling protects me. Now I could feel when someone stepped on my toes. It was as simple as feeling and as challenging as feeling. What a wonderful challenge to have met!

At first, I found it much easier to feel, to be in touch with myself, when I was at home alone. At times, being alone was enjoyable and wonderful. I liked my own company now. Other times, I wanted to be with people. It took me time to gather enough strength to go out and be with people, as the new person I was (the true person I was). I wasn't used to being me in this world. But now, I had a basis — I had me and I knew who *me* was. Even so, venturing out into the world was like this:

I had turned off all the lights. I sat on the floor in the middle of my bedroom meditating, legs crossed. There were no sounds, no distractions. I could feel myself breathe. I could feel my energy vibrate in my body. I could hear my thoughts. I could picture bubbles flowing down the river and could respond to them. I was with me, my thoughts and my feelings. I could feel my spirit, a loving presence. All was so peaceful. Right then, I knew who I was and how I felt. I felt happy.

Yet among all this peacefulness, I felt like something was missing. I wanted to share myself with others. I wanted to laugh, joke, talk and do things with other people. So I stood up, left the room, and went out to a party I had been invited to. Fifty people filled the party room with laughter, loud conversation and blaring music. To communicate, one had to yell over the music. I greeted many of my friends. My peace and tranquility had long been forgotten. My own vibrations had been overridden. I was vibrating all right — the music was blasting.

Half an hour after I got there, I realized that I had lost touch with myself. I left the room, went to the washroom and took a deep breath. Slowly, as I continued to breathe, I regained the peace and my own vibration. I looked in the mirror, smiled at myself, and felt happy again. I went back to the party room and really began to enjoy myself. I was being me. I was no longer vibrating to everyone else's tune.

It was a continual challenge not to vibrate to the tune of others during the following months, while I was reintegrating into society. I had been doing it for 29 years. Reorienting to my own vibrations was a constant effort. When I let up on that effort even a little, I lost touch with myself. I had to remain centred. I had to keep asking myself what I wanted, needed, felt or desired.

Staying centred on me meant I had to keep my focus on me. Since focusing on others had been my life's work, focusing on me was uncomfortable. Yet, it was exactly what I wanted to do. Many times during this process, I was afraid to honour myself. What if I say or do the wrong thing? Then I'd ask myself: "What will happen if I say or do the wrong thing? What is the wrong thing? And what will happen if I honour me?" The answer: the real consequence of honouring, respecting and living as me was being happy and fulfilled. The consequence of doing the opposite was living as I had been for so many years, as a puppet to the rest of the world, contributing nothing as myself. It was still challenging.

By the fourth year of recovery, I felt ready to more fully function in the world. I felt safe and protected by my boundary, my sense of self. I ventured out, while protecting my mind, body and spirit.

I had my own mind. I had my own thoughts. I had my own way of learning. I had difficulty learning many things — I knew that I had an intellect. When my friend at the restaurant told me that my choice of words was improper, he was mistaken, not me. If I had not known what I had meant to say, I might have believed him and taken his criticism as true. I might have thought that I was wrong, dumb and unable to choose the proper words. But I wasn't wrong or dumb and I hadn't chosen improper words. However, what was most important was that his words did not get past my mental boundary.

When he was speaking, his words stayed around him, they didn't reach me. I pictured his words contained in a bubble extending from his mouth, like in a cartoon strip. Although his words had shocked me, I didn't take them into myself or feel personally attacked by them. Instead, I thought: "Wow, he must be down or sad." What was even more inspiring to me, was that I was able to spar with my girlfriend about his inaccurate words. I knew what I meant. My words were mine — his were his. I had a mental boundary.

I wanted to learn more about how boundaries were crossed, so I became an observer. I watched and listened as people communicated with each other. I heard so much boundary crossing. I heard: "You can't do that! You don't think that, do you? What's wrong with you? You dummy. That was stupid!" When I watched television, I noticed verbal cuts and sarcastic remarks on just about every program. I also recognized body language. A facial expression spoke louder than any words. Rolled eyes, shaking heads or pursed lips could tell someone they were a dummy more effectively than any words. When someone spoke and pointed a finger, I pictured their words travelling right back up their finger and arm. I watched and I learned.

I quickly learned that other people have a mind, body and spirit, just as I do. People have beliefs, messages, hurts and fears, just as I do. Every time I spoke, thought or acted, I revealed myself. I revealed my hurt, my fear, my joy and my perceptions. (Sometimes I wondered if all the communications in the world weren't just everyone's projection of their own hurt, fear and joy.) I once heard a saying: "You can't squeeze strawberry juice from a grapefruit." I give to the world what I have inside me.

My greatest challenge was keeping my messages outside my boundary. Often thoughts which were most often messages, would fill my head, inside my boundary. Discarding them was the challenge. Sometimes I just couldn't get away from them. They were like hundreds of flies buzzing around me. I found myself most challenged when I was in the shower in the morning. I would think about what I had said to someone, what I would say when I met them again, what I had done the previous day and what I hadn't done.

Some days it was easy to say to myself: "I'm not going to spend my time and energy focused on that thought about that person." Other days, I spent time obsessing about what a mere acquaintance had said to me. Sometimes my thoughts helped me work out a situation or a relationship with someone and resolve it so I could attain peace of mind.

But, until I reached a resolution, I would spent a great deal of time thinking about those thoughts. The worst were the messages that didn't come from outside, but had been inside my boundary for many years. Now, I had the prerogative to choose which ones I wanted to think about and respond to and which ones I didn't.

To do this, I needed to stop what I was doing, take some quiet time (sometimes only a few minutes) and ask myself whether I wanted to continue thinking about it or not. (Deep breathing helped a lot.) Sometimes I would let out a visceral yell and then feel much better. If I didn't let go of a bothersome thought and let it flow down the river, it could drive me crazy for hours. All my time, effort, focus and energy wasted on a thought! Thoughts disrupted my peace. I could honour my boundary, my peace of mind, open my boundary door and let my thought go.

I wanted to shout "no!" from the treetops. All those years when something happened that I didn't want, I had swallowed my "no." Now, when I didn't want something, I said no. And it felt so good. (I felt like the young kid finally being able to say no to the powerful parent. I felt the anger, energy and frustration release.) When my friend asked me to go to lunch and I said no, not wanting to go, I felt good. When I said no to a job I didn't want, I felt good. When I said no to a man who wanted something I didn't, I felt good. I was protecting myself. I was so happy. I felt safe. I trusted myself. I was honouring myself. I had a boundary. I was not willing to sacrifice myself, my feelings or my integrity ever again. I would not do something I didn't want to. I wasn't dependent anymore. I wasn't willing to play the game any longer — I'll do this for you if you do that for me.

I learned to communicate my wants and needs gently and clearly. Some people had different perspectives and different boundaries than mine. Sometimes describing what I wanted without offending someone was difficult. Unfortunately, communicating my needs and wants was necessary. Usually when I expressed my want or need, the person understood and honoured my wishes. Other times, I found that I was repeating myself or justifying my position. As soon as I realized that I was justifying, I stopped and removed myself from the situation. Some people will do as they please, regardless of the consequences to others. I can't change other people, but I can change my position. I can remove myself from a situation or person. I can make my own necessary changes. I can protect me.

The world is full of feedback. I received negative as well as positive feedback. I found it extremely difficult to handle negative feedback from a person who really mattered to me. I had to put their words into proper perspective. Honouring my boundary with my friend at the restaurant was easier than with a man, friend or family member. The world is full of people who actively share their opinions and ideas. Some people express their ideas strongly. I was determined to be me.

I was driving down the road when I looked into my rear view mirror and saw the front of a blue Mustang, just feet away from my back bumper. I felt aggravated so I sped up. Before I knew it, I was speeding, without having ever intended to. The guy in the Mustang must have been in a rush because he kept trying to pass me, but there was too much traffic. Then, he hit the gas and bolted out from behind me. Then he cut in front of me! I thought: "What did I ever do to him? Was I driving too slowly?" I knew I wasn't. (Interestingly, my first thought was that I had caused him to drive that way.) I was now speeding at 20 miles per hour above the speed limit.

Finally he was out of sight, but I was fuming. Why had I let this guy drive me so crazy? I could have been pulled over and given a speeding ticket. I felt frustrated and disappointed with myself. I hadn't wanted to speed but I had responded to his actions, not mine. Feeling angry, I decided right then and there that I would never let another driver affect my speed of travel. I had let that guy get to me, cross my boundary — but never again. (I had to reach a point of great frustration and anger to realize my boundary; but I did it!) I drive very calmly now. When someone wants to pass me, or honks their horn at me, they can keep on honking. I keep on driving.

I knew I was sensitive to other people's energy and I made an extra effort to appreciate my sensitivity. I tried hard not to respond to a person's mood, speed or vibration. I had many opportunities to practise. I had a friend who spoke at a rate of three hundred words a minute. I no longer tried to keep up. Sometimes, if a person was silent, I'd be silent too. No longer. I decided to live at my own speed, which might be quite different to that of the person I was with. If I felt like joking, I'd joke. If a friend was making one joke after another, and I didn't feel like joking, I'd just laugh. I no longer felt the need to be at the same level as the person I was with. What a relief!

I protected my body. My body is mine. People can look at it and make faces. But ultimately, what did it all mean? Who feeds my body? Me. Who exercises my body? Me. Who clothes my body? Me. Who feels my body? Me. Who breathes in oxygen? Me. How does a person walking down the road affect my body? They don't. How many hours a day does someone else live in my body? None. Then why on earth have I spent so much time making my body right for everyone else — but me? No longer! I now spend time making my body right for me.

My outfit that day was not "interesting," as my friend so eloquently put it. I liked it. It was different, fun, and quite conservatively funky. I felt good in it because it was an expression of me. Everyone has their own taste.

It took me what seemed like forever to realize this a simple truth — the way a person responds to my body reveals who they are. A person's acceptance or rejection of my body has no consequences for my survival.

I had starved myself. I could blame society for my starving and purging because of the pressure it places on women to be thin. But, blaming won't change anything. True, society does place high value on a good body, but why should this be so? I'm not my body. Love doesn't come from the body. Laughter doesn't come from the body. Talent doesn't come from the body. Intelligence doesn't come from the body. I believe that the body is definitely overrated.

The day I was walking to the restaurant, men were looking at my body. Some men looked more closely than others. I don't know exactly what they were thinking, but I can guess. I can't stop people from thinking their thoughts, but I can remove my own discomfort. I dress quite conservatively; I don't reveal my body to strangers. I protect my body by covering it. I do not want to be the object of a man's fantasy. The key word here is *object*. I know that when a man is attracted to my body, getting to know me is the last thing on his mind. I am not interested in relating to anyone on a level other than love, honesty and good communication.

I watch the interaction between men and women. I realized that we humans have natural instincts. I realize that a woman attracts a man, and then they can mate. What I don't understand is why a man or woman would have their picture taken with their clothes off for the entire world to see. I guess each of us has different boundaries. I would not be proud of myself if I had done that. Attention is not equal. There is quality attention, and there is not. A man's sexual desire has nothing to do with love. I protect my body by allowing someone to touch it in a way that is pleasing to me. I remove myself from the company of a person who does not honour what is okay for me.

One day, I was having a discussion with a group of women. We had been talking, laughing and having a great time when, out of the blue, I asked them: "Does our body size affect our enjoyment right now?" We all looked at each other and said: "No, the size of our body does not touch our hearts." I have never loved socializing or laughing with a person's body. It's the heart that touches me. I have appreciated and enjoyed looking at a well-toned body. I have never been in love with biceps and quadriceps.

I protected my spirit. I was sensitive to the feelings of others. I cared about what people liked, disliked, felt and wanted. Telling someone something that I knew would be disappointing or saddening was so difficult for me, especially someone I cared about. Unfortunately, it was necessary at times. I had to honour me.

I communicated how I felt to the people I truly cared for. If I liked something, I expressed my like. If I didn't, I expressed that too. I was honouring myself, yet doing so brought with it some fear. I was afraid of the consequence of telling someone that I didn't like what they were doing. I was afraid to tell someone that I was not willing to continue what I had been doing. I was afraid that the person would leave me.

I found it especially hard to describe my lack of feeling to a man who cared for me, who hoped for a future together. Describing how I felt to my family members was the hardest of all. Yet, at times, I knew that I had to, especially if someone had said or had done something that hurt me. Sometimes I would get so angry, I would have to first walk away from the situation, and then put my anger into perspective.

I knew that my anger was a reaction to a perceived boundary crossing and that made me afraid. Once I understood the cause of my fear, I could tell the person. I shared my feelings most of the time. Sometimes, sharing would not have made a positive difference. Sometimes, sharing my feelings only set me up for someone to try to cross my boundary again. I shared my feelings when it felt right. I listened to my boundary, my gut reaction.

Now, I clearly understood that for many years, I held onto the inaccurate belief that I caused others their pain. I realized that it was quite self-centred to believe that I was the cause of everyone's response. I never stopped to ask myself if I really had the power to make people happy, sad, angry or crazy. Now I understood that their reactions were about them, not me. I felt a huge burden lift. No one was responsible for my feelings.

I was not responsible for theirs. Guilt trips were no longer possible. I didn't feel guilty for a person's pain. I wished that they didn't have to feel pain, but I knew that pain was part of life. I also knew that pain was survivable. After all, I was still here.

I no longer felt so sensitive. I didn't feel shame for expressing my emotions. I realized that when a person told me to get over it, that I was overreacting, and making more out of something than need be, that they were actually revealing themselves. Their words were theirs.

Everyone has a different perspective on life. I try not to judge others. Nor do I feel the need to respond to the judgement of others. When my friend told me that my words were "improper," I could have taken his judgement personally and reworded my sentences. My words were not improper. My words were mine. His judgement was his.

He didn't like my outfit. That didn't mean it was unattractive, only that he didn't like it. I did. Two separate preferences. I realized that a person's preferences in life vary as much as a their taste in food. No two people like all the same foods (no two people I have met). No two people like all the same hobbies. No two people always think the same way or always feel the same way. I believe that everyone is equal. I also believe that everyone is different. Some differences are greater than others. Some differences are compatible and some are not, but they are differences all the same, not meant for people to judge.

Living in this world, with others, each of us with our own unique differences, offered me a huge challenge. I was challenged to stand tall and stay true to myself. Living with so many other people telling me what to say, what to do, how to live, required that I honour, respect and most of all, live as me. I was challenged to reach inside myself and find out what I wanted. I was not interested in living out the likes, preferences, wishes and ideals of other people. I was determined to live as me.

At times, I found it challenging to keep my focus and carry out my own wishes, especially when a person I cared for strongly disagreed. The world was loud, offering many obstacles to peacefulness. The world was obnoxious at times. The world was harsh in its judgements. But, the world was also beautiful, loving and enjoyable. I wanted to live as part of the world. I decided to take the good with the bad.

I was about to give life to my thoughts, dreams, inspiration and wishes. I was about to make them real. I was about to initiate activities that I had only dreamed about a short time ago. I was ready to express myself.

Twenty-Three

I
TRIED
MY BEST

Age 29

I was lying in bed early one morning, contemplating life. I had so many drives, so many desires. I wanted to be a seamstress. I wanted to design and make my own clothes. I could picture the colours, cuts and fabrics of my designs. I wanted to sing and spend hours lost in the rhythms of music. I wanted to write my own songs. I wanted to cut hair and give seminars about fashion, beauty and style. Most of all, I wanted to give seminars on eating disorders. There were so many things I wanted to do. As I lay there, I felt certain that I could do all of those things, and more. I just didn't know how to get started.

I felt as though a huge mountain stood between thinking about my desires and acting on them. Thinking about the endless possibilities of life was fun, but contemplating the process of learning how to implement them instantly destroyed the excitement. Every time I thought about actually doing something, I felt shame. It was now time to look my shame message: "I can't do anything right" in the face. Trying had always been so painful. I had failed at so many things. I recalled the laughter when I tried to draw. I remembered the ridicule when I tried to sing. Being laughed at and ridiculed was so painful that I vowed that unless I did something perfectly from the beginning, I would never do it. Unfortunately, I heeded that vow and tried very little as a result.

Until now, I had no idea that when people begin something new, they rarely do it perfectly. I hadn't considered that most people make many mistakes when learning something new. Now, I was going to try to sew. I had wanted to do this for several years now. Now the shame, fear and doubt could not keep me from trying. I understood that the roots of those emotions were the messages I carried. Faulty messages had stood in my way for far too long now. I was no longer willing to let them get in the way of my life anymore.

I hopped out of bed and circled my sewing machine. I had owned it for the last 30 days and it was sitting in the middle of my dining room table. I had resolved not to dine at the table until I tried to sew. I walked past the machine many times a day. I was trying to warm up to my machine, almost like it was human.

I was feeling less and less afraid of using it as the days passed. I had gone to stores to look at how clothes were sewn. Yesterday, I had worked up the nerve to go to the store where I bought the machine and ask for a basic lesson on how to use it. Now today, this morning, I plugged it in. I had fabric and a pattern. I opened the pattern, glanced at all the writing in what seemed like foreign language and quickly stuffed it back into the package. I was afraid. I was sure I wouldn't be able to understand it.

I felt overwhelmingly shameful. I got into the shower and began to cry. I wanted so much to be able to sew but just didn't have the confidence that I could do it. After a few minutes I stopped crying and felt calmer. The feeling of extreme shame had dissipated with my tears. I stepped out of the shower, got dressed and went back to the machine. One again, I took out the pattern. I thought to myself: "Someone drew these shapes and wrote down these instructions. I can read, so I will be able to understand it." Still I could feel a gnawing shame (now at volume two, not ten).

I took a deep breath and appealed to my guardian angel for help: "Please help me read this pattern!" I looked at the shapes and pieces of a jumpsuit, feeling no longer alone, thinking to myself how I had always wanted someone who loved me to be with me when I tried something new. I was surprised to find that the pattern and its instructions were really quite straightforward. I cut my fabric according to the instructions. I had the proper thread and accessories to begin sewing.

I put the first two pieces together, put my foot on the pedal and pushed down. The sewing machine began to work. I followed the line along the seam and came to the end. I removed the fabric and opened it to see what it looked like. I couldn't believe it. The outfit appeared to be sewn properly, the same way as clothes in stores were. I was so happy. I could barely contain myself. I kept sewing until two hours had passed and I had finished the jumpsuit.

I had cried, sweated and somehow continued to try, and kept on sewing. I had overcome the frustration, anxiety and doubts I experienced in those hours and the preceding weeks. I had completed my first outfit! I felt like I was on top of the world.

At the time, I didn't know what gave me the courage to persevere with sewing, through so much fear of failing. A part of me knew that if other people could sew, so could I. Making that jumpsuit was my first accomplishment since beginning my recovery one and a half years before. Today, two and a half years later, I can make almost anything my sewing machine can handle. But, I know I'd never be in this position if I hadn't taken the first step and tried.

Doubt was my only real obstacle, an obstacle that had prevented me from making my thoughts, dreams and desires come true. Doubt was what kept me from creating and expressing myself. I wish I could have just gotten rid of my doubt and been able to get on with what I wanted to do. However, my doubt was present, until I faced it, felt it and saw it for what it was — false. I had proven my doubt wrong. I could sew. I kept at it even when my doubt was at its strongest.

I had to try very hard to remember that my doubt was a message that could be put outside my boundary. I pictured myself with my luminous circle around me and the message of doubt in a bubble floating outside of it, hitting up against my boundary. I could let that message come inside and listen to it or leave it outside where it belonged. I had listened to these destructive messages long enough. Also, I reminded myself of a saying when I felt afraid to try: My doubts are traitors; they will win, if I listen to them and don't try.

The next thing I tried was to do was write a song. Again, I felt over-whelmed with doubts just thinking about trying. Yet in the strongest way, I knew I could do it. I had wanted to write songs for years now. I couldn't believe how terribly painful my doubts were. They were like voices in my head coming from all angles around me which just kept coming. I felt like I was going crazy! No one was around me yet I was hearing voices — voices of others and my own. Before I reached what felt like insanity, I shouted: "Stop! You're not going to get to me!"

I took a huge breath and looked up to my angel, pleading for help. I closed my eyes and pictured myself on the shore watching my doubts float down the river. There they were: You can't do it; you don't have it in you; no one will listen; don't bother, people will only laugh; don't even try, you'll just fail again. I couldn't believe what was floating by me. None of it was true, but the words and their meanings were incredibly powerful.

These were some of the thoughts I used to counter my doubts: "So what if I don't write the perfect song? What really, is the consequence of that? What does failure really mean? What is failure anyway? What is the consequence of failing? One part of me said: "Well, I might be a failure at writing songs and it's something I really want to do. "Really?" questioned another. "Will writing one less-than-perfect song mean that I've failed at it? Does that mean that I won't ever be able to write songs?" "Well, no, I guess...Well, no, I guess not!"

I realized then that I could learn to write songs the way most other people do. I could read an instructional book and learn the basic format of songwriting. I could talk to songwriters. Yet, my fear of feeling the pain of failure had been enough to prevent me from trying. My fear of feeling the pain of failure was the consequence of trying. But was failure happening right now? No. I hadn't even tried yet. So how did I know that I was going to fail?

All I came up with was a feeling, a fearful feeling from the past, from a long-carried message. I experienced that pain years ago, when I was criticized by others. No one was around me, yet I had the feeling there was. I feared that someone was bound to criticize what I was about to do. I asked myself how criticism mattered to me now. It didn't. Yes, I am still sensitive to criticism, but it doesn't pierce me in the same way.

I have a boundary now and I know that when a person is critical, they reveal more about themselves than me. Now, instead of criticism being painful, giving up is painful. I can try and try and try, and do my best. I can learn, I know I have the capability. I can write the best song I can, only if I try. If I give up, and give in to my inaccurate doubt, I will truly fail. Also, I will fail to know what I might have been. Not trying is failure.

I looked up to my angel and said: "Thank you. I will try my best to write a song." There are no consequences to trying. I refused to give my fear of failing, my doubts, or my messages any power over me any longer. I stopped listening to them, right at that moment. I began to write a song.

I had a vision — a mental picture — of what I wanted to do before I actually did it. Without the vision, I only got frustrated. Now, if I'm feeling frustrated, I ask myself: "What do I want to do?" and then try to picture it. If I can't picture it, I don't do it. I could picture the finished jumpsuit before I started sewing. I could picture the finished song, the verses, the chorus and the section eight, before I started writing. Sometimes, it took a while for me to develop a clear vision. But when I was patient and waited until I had one, doing things was simple. When I did things without one, I'd end up spinning my wheels and going in circles, getting frustrated. Sometimes, all I needed was a format to work within, like writing a song. I didn't have to know the words, I could create within a framework. I was always successful when I could picture a final product or picture myself doing it.

I went through a four-phase cycle (a circle divided into quarters) every time I accomplished something. This seemed to me a bit like a washing machine, after four cycles, my accomplishment would come out clean. I had a starting point, a quarter-way challenge, a half-way inspiration, a three-quarter-way challenge and then completion.

I wanted to write this book. When I began, I didn't know how to write a book — a long report had been challenge enough. Yet, I could envision the book. I felt inspired from deep within me. I was motivated, excited and absolutely certain that this book would take form. I began to make my vision real. I wrote the outline of the chapters. Then I expanded it four times, until I had one page per chapter. Then I chose a chapter, and fleshed it out. I would put almost everything I wanted to say in the book in that one chapter.

I wasn't at all knowledgable about how to write a book. (If I could look back at what I wrote, I'd be shocked that I kept going.) My writing was terrible; I didn't know how to do it. I didn't know the basics of writing, structure or grammar. Up until I reached my first reality checkpoint — the first quarter-way challenge, I wrote from inspiration alone. That challenge felt like hitting a brick wall. I had travelled a quarter of the way through without realizing that I didn't have enough knowledge or skill to proceed. I really felt stupid. I felt stupid for having come this far, to even think that *I* could write a book. I wondered how I had gotten myself into this position in the first place. I felt so much pressure, awkwardness and frustration. I didn't know where to turn. I wanted so badly to run as fast, and as far away, as possible from writing this book. I hadn't told many people about the book, and I was grateful for that. I wouldn't have to be too embarrassed when I inevitably failed to produce it. I could just hear the gossip: "I knew she couldn't do it. Have you seen Sheila's book on the shelf? I don't know where she got the idea that she could write a book."

But, as much as I wanted to run from my responsibility, something inside kept pushing me to keep going. I felt as though I were being prompted to walk into the deep end of a pool. My head was about to go under water. And I was determined to learn how to swim. I went to the bookstore and bought three books. One was how to write, one was on grammar, and the third was on how to express from within. I read each word. I spend hours sweating over that information. I was intent on learning how. Before I realized it, I had long forgotton my doubts about the book, and was writing again.

This time, I had a foundation of knowledge to write from. I could have thrown up my hands at the first quarter phase, but I didn't. I was happily writing. I would begin early in the morning on some days. I would write late into the night on others — the night was such a peaceful time to work. Once I resumed writing, I was so happy that I had learned how to keep going.

I thought that it was clear sailing from there — that I had hit the only barrier. I had been writing for months when I reached the half-way point and everything seemed so clear. I could envision the book in its completed form. I could see the order of the chapters. I thoroughly enjoyed this point with its insight and inspiration. Filled with energy and excitement, I wrote for many more months. Then I read an article in a magazine stating that the average writer re-writes a manuscript 14 times. I was feeling quite relieved — I had rewritten mine at least that many times.

By this time, I had reached the three-quarter phase — the most challenging one. I was 75 percent completed when the feelings of doubt, shame and fear overwhelmed me. I felt incapable of writing properly, underqualified to write a book and afraid of failing. I was ridden with self-doubt. I went to the side of the river and faced those doubts. It was painfully challenging to keep going, even thought I was almost finished. By this time, I had told lots of people about my book. Everyone had their questions: When is it going to be finished? Do you have a publisher? What education do you have? Do you know how difficult it is to get a book published these days?

I felt like an open book! I really had to exert my boundary. I pictured myself inside my boundary and the others inside theirs. When someone was critical, I would envision their words travelling right back up their finger and arm. (So many people point!) I was determined not to resonate to their negative vibrations. After being inundated with critical questions, I'd tell the person that I had things covered, and walk away. But, underneath it all, I also felt uneasy about those questions.

Somehow, however, I felt confident that things would happen as they were supposed to. I kept writing. I borrowed books on publishing and editing from the library and felt more confident after reading them. I continued through my last phase. I was on the downhill stretch, approaching completion. After having tuned out the world and focusing completely on my work, I finished the book! I had come full circle. I had done it! I had persevered and achieved my vision.

Every time I completed something, I was ecstatic. Large and small accomplishments gave me the same euphoric feeling. I felt equal satisfaction from sewing my first jumpsuit, writing my first song and writing this book. I did it, despite what people said! I followed my heart. I applied myself, worked through all my doubts and made it. My self-confidence and self-esteem were growing. I was showing myself that no matter the challenge, trying was what mattered. The quality of the result was irrelevant. I stopped rating what I had done. There was no scale of one to 10 anymore. My effort was my scale. Applying 100% effort rated a 10. Accepting less than perfection was new. I knew that if I wanted to, I could always do better, by trying, learning and practising. The more I tried and succeeded in completing something, the more inspired I was to try other things. I tried many.

Understanding that there were obstacles, barriers and challenges associated with everything I tried helped to propel me through them. I could anticipate barriers and knew that they were a natural part of the process. Sometimes when I experienced those barriers, I would feel angry, and sometimes that anger was just the energy I needed to keep going.

Experiencing those barriers often prompted me to take lessons or classes at school. I realized there were times when I couldn't find out the answers or learn how to do something by myself. Previously, I had been too afraid to take instruction from someone because I was afraid of failing and looking bad in the eyes of someone else. On the first day I took singing lessons, the teacher asked me to sing the C major scale. I turned beet-red as this sound, like a squeak, came out of my mouth. I was mortified. I knew I could do *much* better than that. I wished I could have crawled under the piano she was playing.

I swallowed what felt like a grader, looked my teacher in the eye and told her I was nervous and not used to singing in front of people. She smiled and said: "Don't worry, every one is afraid at first. I've heard all kinds of voices. We'll make yours sound beautiful." I took a deep breath, sang the scale, and knew that I had some practising to do. She showed me how to breathe and position my body. I went home and practised and practised. The people from whom I took my singing, astrology, and college classes were truly compassionate teachers. I felt no condemnation from them, although I made many mistakes. They were interested in effort, not results. And I was trying!

I took tennis lessons, singing lessons, astrology courses and business courses. I wanted to learn and learn and learn. I loved the feeling I had when I accomplished something. I knew now that an accomplishment required great effort and hard work. A doctor is not born knowing anatomy. It takes many years of study to become a doctor. I hadn't really thought about the process of beginning something; spending time, effort and energy learning it; and then doing it. I did not appreciate the great effort required to become a doctor, a professional tennis player or singer. I would try to sing and if I couldn't do it as well as Whitney Houston or Mariah Carey, I would quit, thinking I couldn't do it. I didn't understand that comparing my voice to those well-trained and highly practised voices was quite unrealistic. If I had spent as much time as they had on practising and lessons, then a comparison might have been reasonable. Even so, my voice is my voice. It is different from anyone else's. Now, I just practise singing and enjoy my own sound. It isn't the best and it isn't the worst. It's pleasant, it's mine and I like it.

Some things came more easily than others. Sometimes I would have difficulty understanding the information or instructions in books. Yet, I knew that if a person could write it, I could understand it. I chuckle now, but I used to think that the text in newspapers, magazines and books was written by some kind of genius machine. It never occurred to me that an ordinary person wrote those words. And if I didn't understand what the words meant, then there was something wrong with me. Sometimes a book or article was poorly written, or I just had difficulty understanding it. I knew that I processed information in my own way. People can learn aurally, visually and/or kinetically. Books are visual. It took me time to learn how to assimilate the words from books to formulate a picture. With great effort and practice, I could do it. I hadn't read many books by the time I was twenty. Sometimes I understood information and other times I didn't, but I tried my best.

Accomplishing things took time. It took time for me to sing well. It took time for me to sew well. It took time for me to learn astrology. I took lessons and worked hard at what I was trying to do. Sometimes the work was frustrating, sometimes it was aggravating and sometimes it was a lot of fun. When I spent the time and effort and tried my best, I always felt happy. Happiness was my reward. Happiness was growth. I grew and grew.

Finally, I was trying many of the things I'd always wanted to try. There are still some that I hadn't yet tried, but I know I can only do so much. There's a part of me that wants to try them all — now. I can be like a starving kid at a buffet table, sure to load my plate beyond my capacity. I have to practise patience.

Continuing to persevere, when the people around me were pessimistic and unsupportive, was challenging. I chose to be only with supportive people and I practised my boundary. Some days I spent alone, other days I spent with people. Sometimes I travelled, other times I stayed at home. Most of all, my days were filled with joy. Frustrations and challenges were also a part of my life. Experiencing sorrow helped me to cherish joy even more. I experienced the joy of accomplishment when I overcame challenges and difficulties to reach that accomplishment. I rarely celebrated when things came easily. I live with joy, peace, sorrow and challenge. I'm here on earth to grow, to learn, and to feel. I was living.

Twenty-Four

LEAVING
FOOD
BEHIND

Age 30

I *woke up on a beautiful summer morning and leapt out of bed. I felt a drive to live! The past was behind me. I felt no need to cling to it or change it in any way. Today was a new day with new choices. I could do what I wanted. I looked forward to new challenges. What other people thought had no bearing on my choices. I went downstairs, poured myself a cup of coffee, and sat outside on my backyard deck.*

As I stood up to look out over the park that extended from my backyard, I was actually looking back to where I had come from, the past four years of my recovery. Now, I felt happy and peaceful with life and with my place in it. I watched the the birds busily building their nest. I watched the grace and form of the geese in flight passing just over me. My thoughts returned to me. I smiled, feeling such joy, I had attained a firm foundation within myself.

I liked who I was. I wanted to be all that I was. I was eager to live life. I was ready. I knew that there would be times I would feel overwhelmed with fear. I knew that shame would always be a part of my life. I knew that I'd experience pain and disappointment, probably many times. But joy and love were at the centre of my thoughts. I had hope. I had excitement. Negative thoughts no longer ruled, although they were still present.

I knew that it was time for me to fulfill my purpose in life but I didn't have a clear definition of what that was. I did know that I was to live life with love, guided by my feelings and my spiritual guide. I was just beginning to live the life that had always been mine. I went into the house to prepare. I had some catching up to do.

I began my recovery more than five years ago. More than four years ago, I had been bulimic, and was overeating or starving myself. On that morning, I had awakened feeling peaceful and happy. I had grieved my past, and now I could move on. I had my whole life ahead of me.

I saw so many opportunities for me to experience joy, sorrow, challenge and love. I knew that my life on earth had a purpose. I knew that there had been a reason that I experienced an eating disorder and recovered from it. I knew that I would not know myself to this degree without having had that experience. I understood that every experience had a purpose.

I felt as though I had stepped out of from under a heavy black cloud that had enveloped me throughout my recovery. I wasn't sorry about anything that had happened or resentful toward anyone. I felt joy deep within my heart. The black cloud was behind me now, hovering over the mountain through which I had just portaged.

Unfortunately, I still had fear. I still had shame and I still had pain. I still had negative internal messages, and will until I die. But, now I chose to converse with those messages, rather than give up my precious energy to them. I didn't always know what message was affecting me instantaneously. I didn't always have the answer about how to go on when I felt something strongly. Yet, I did know that as long as I stopped what I was doing and conversed with my emotion, I could proceed. Sometimes I cried right then and there. Sometimes I let out a good visceral yell. But I always allowed myself to experience the emotion.

I live with honesty. I live with integrity. I live with happiness. I feel at peace with myself and the world around me. I rejoice with my guardian angel many times a day. I know the spirit world is always close. I still get angry. I still yell. But now I also laugh. I play. I eat when I'm hungry. I feel at peace with my past. I love my parents, brothers and sisters. I'm happy that I grew up in the environment I did. I'm grateful for all the experiences I've had. I am the person I am today because of all of them.

I have left food behind.

Leaving
Food
Behind

Please send a copy of *Leaving Food Behind* to:

Name _____

Address _____

City/Town _____

Province/State _____

Postal Code/Zip Code _____

Telephone _____

Fax _____

How did you hear about the book? _____

_____

When did you hear about the book? _____

_____

Comments _____

_____

Please include a cheque or money order for **$17.99 Cdn** or **$15.89 US**
($14.95 + 1.05 GST + 1.99 S&h Cdn)
($12.95 + .91 GST + 2.03 S&h US)

To order by phone **1 888-572-2135**
(between 8 am-5 pm EST)
(allow 4-6 weeks for delivery)
VISA and MASTERCARD accepted

Mail to: **Mather Publications**
P.O. Box 84031, Pinecrest
Ottawa, ON
K2C 3Z2 Canada

About the Author

SHEILA MATHER is currently providing Seminars on Eating Disorders. Although living in Nepean, Ontario, Canada, Sheila can be found travelling throughout North America, visiting radio and television stations, community centres and schools. Sheila is committed to increasing the awareness of Eating Disorders.

229461